FUNDAMENTALS OF RADIATION THERAPY

FUNDAMENTALS OF RADIATION THERAPY
and Cancer Chemotherapy

SIDNEY LOWRY MD

Professor of Cancer Studies, The Queen's University of Belfast

formerly Director of Radiation Therapy, Maine Medical Center, Portland, Maine
Assistant Professor of Therapeutic Radiology, Tufts-New England
Medical Center, Boston

THE ENGLISH UNIVERSITIES PRESS LTD

FᏎF

ISBN 0 340 18198 2 Boards
ISBN 0 340 18197 4 Paper

First printed 1974

The English Universities Press Ltd
St Paul's House, Warwick Lane, London EC4P 4AH

Printed and bound in Great Britain by
T. & A. Constable Ltd, Edinburgh

Foreword

by **J. F. Fowler,** DSc, PhD, MSc, FInstP

Director of the Gray Laboratory of the Cancer Research Campaign, Mount Vernon Hospital, Northwood, London

This compact book will appeal to a wide variety of readers concerned with cancer treatment. It is much more than an excellent introduction for therapeutic radiologists. It will be a valuable reference book for surgeons, physicians, and other specialists. It will also be of interest to nurses, non-medical laboratory workers and research scientists. Others who deal with patients will be able to obtain a clear perspective of the prospects for the patient offered by radiotherapy in various types of cancer. The author sees a 'pattern of cancer control emerging which involves the whole of medicine'.

Modern techniques can achieve 90 per cent cure rates in Stage I of many types of cancer; but most medical curricula give the subject of radiotherapy scant attention. This book will do much to repair the omission.

The author is a distinguished radiotherapist with broad clinical and scientific experience and interests in cancer research as well. He has produced an admirably readable book, in which the reader can find relevant information easily.

Acknowledgements

I am indebted to Dr Arnold Lyons and Professor John Vallance-Owen who initially encouraged me to write this book. I should also like to thank many of the students and staff of The Royal Victoria Hospital, Belfast, The New England Medical Center, Boston and The Maine Medical Center, Portland, for their helpful comments and suggestions.

My thanks are also due to Dr Basil Stoll, St Thomas' Hospital, London, Dr Anthony Nias, Glasgow Institute of Radiotherapeutics, Dr Leo Stollbach, Pondville Hospital, Boston, and Professor Emil Frei, Harvard Medical School for permission to publish his graph of the development of chemotherapeutic drugs. I am particularly indebted to Dr Fernando Bloedorn, former President of the American Radium Society, whose influence and example permeates these pages; to Mr Selwyn Taylor for his support and encouragement; and to my friend and associate Dr J. Howard Hannemann who cheerfully reviewed the entire manuscript.

I should also like to thank the many secretaries who typed and re-typed the text, including Teresa Perrino, Rachel Theroux and Hilda Toews.

Lastly I wish to thank my wife Barbara, to whom this book is dedicated, for painstakingly reading and correcting the text from cover to cover.

Contents

	Foreword	v
	Acknowledgements	vi
1	Introduction	1
2	Physical Aspects	4
3	Radiobiological Aspects	15
4	Radiation Pathology	22
5	Therapeutic Aspects	29
6	Skin	42
7	Lip and Oral Cavity	49
8	Ear, Nose and Throat	57
9	Orbit and Salivary Glands	68
10	Central Nervous System	74
11	Endocrine Glands	79
12	Thorax	85
13	Abdomen	91
14	Bone and Soft Tissues	95
15	Lympho-reticular System	103
16	Blood Disorders	112
17	Female Genital Tract	120
18	Male Genital Tract	134
19	The Urinary Tract	138
20	Breast	146
21	Malignant Disease in Childhood and Pregnancy	154

22   Benign Diseases   160
23   Recent Advances   166
24   Cancer Chemotherapy   173
     Index   191

1

Introduction

Cancer is the second main cause of death today. For over 50 years radiotherapy has played a vital part in the treatment and control of this disease. Yet paradoxically little is known about radiotherapy outside the specialty itself. Few textbooks have been written on the subject. Considering the number of books on radiological physics this is surprising.

The present volume has been written mainly as an introduction for students and young physicians who may be contemplating a career in radiotherapy or oncology. At the same time it may be of value to others who would like to know, briefly, what radiation therapy has to offer in a particular clinical situation.

The principles of radiotherapy and their application in clinical practice are discussed. The scope of the book is wide, since radiotherapy has a part to play in almost every medical specialty. I have aimed to be concise; however, a few topics of special interest to the radiotherapist are dealt with in a little more detail. These include Hodgkin's disease and cancer of the cervix. The format generally follows the outline: aetiology, pathology, clinical features, investigations, treatment and results. An attempt has been made to place the subject in its proper context. Where the treatment of choice is surgery, this is stated.

Inevitably in a book of this size, some of the presentation is dogmatic. However, selected references are made to the original literature for those who wish to pursue the subject further.

Five-year survival figures are quoted for most diseases. Where available, absolute cure rates are given. Over 30 per cent of cancer patients are cured; a further 30 to 40 per cent obtain useful and prolonged palliation; the remainder are incurable.

Considerable progress has been made in radiotherapy, especially since the introduction of supervoltage equipment. Survival figures for certain cancer sites treated by radiation show steady improvement over the years. Table I gives figures for 1949 and 1969. It has been pointed out that these improvements were achieved step by step. If we expect too much too quickly we shall feel unnecessarily disappointed. Clinical cancer trials are now under way in many centres. However large numbers of patients—perhaps thousands

TABLE I

Improved survival of several types of cancer over 20 year period

Type of cancer	3-year survival (per cent) 1949	3-year survival (per cent) 1969
Hodgkin's disease	35	61
Cancer of the cervix	53	63
Cancer of the prostate	49	66
Cancer of the nose	30	47
Cancer of the bladder	48	62
Cancer of the skin	49	74
Cancer of the testes	52	69
Cancer of the larynx	41	54

From: *Cancer Research Campaign, London.*

— will have to be followed for many years before small differences in survival can be reliably detected.

A section on cytotoxic drugs is included at the end of the book. The role of the cancer chemotherapist has yet to be clearly defined. In Britain, most cytotoxic therapy is given by the radiotherapist. This has been profitable in many ways. For one thing, radiotherapy is a form of chemotherapy, and cytotoxic side effects resemble radiation damage. In the USA, however, the bulk of cancer chemotherapy is given by the internist or general physician. Medical oncologists, as they have come to be known, have a background in general medicine and therapeutics with additional training in cytotoxic therapy. At present, however, chemotherapy is still in its infancy, and the clinician should not shrink from offering radical surgery or radical radiotherapy where indicated. Inadequate surgery plus inadequate radiotherapy adds up to inadequate treatment, and a compromise with cancer leads only to defeat.

Looking to the future, it seems likely that the answer to cancer will come from many different disciplines. Malignant disease may, in fact, be controlled in much the same way as tuberculosis. It will be recalled that tuberculosis was largely eradicated, not by streptomycin alone, but also by better social conditions, mass X-ray, skin testing, BCG and so on.

Today mule-spinners' cancer of the scrotum has been eradicated. Industrial cancer of the bladder is uncommon. Soap and water have practically eliminated carcinoma of the penis. Education could make lung carcinoma a rare disease. One can begin to see a pattern of control emerging which involves the whole of medicine.

The management of cancer of the cervix emphasizes this multidisciplinary approach. Simple hygiene has lowered the incidence of the disease. Developments in cytology have perfected the pap smear test. Social and preventive medicine have made the test available to large numbers of people. Education has increased public awareness. Epidemiology has identified the patients at risk. Surgery can eradicate pre-invasive carcinoma-in-situ. Modern radio-therapeutic techniques have provided up to 90 per cent cure rates in Stage I disease. Even in advanced disease, the use of the multimillion volt betatron has produced excellent results.

So curiously, here we have a situation where an important form of cancer is being effectively controlled and may even be wiped out in our lifetime and these developments have had little to do with a 'magic bullet' or injection. Indeed it might be said that the main problem in carcinoma of the cervix today, is the grand multiparous woman of the lower socioeconomic group who totally neglects herself until she has incurable disease. This is a problem. And it is an important problem. But it is not a problem for molecular biology.

The above approach may not seem an ambitious programme but it is a realistic one, for the problem of cancer is as involved as the problem of growth itself. Furthermore, it has been stated with some authority that we will not learn much more about malignant growth until we know more about normal growth.

In addition a number of patients with advanced cancer are learning to live with their disease. This is not a nihilistic approach. Diabetes cannot be cured but it can be controlled with insulin. The same is true for some forms of cancer.

Meanwhile the immediate problem of patient management remains, and we must consolidate the gains already made. Most medical curricula give the subject of radiotherapy scant attention. Not long ago, a medical student in his final year remarked that he was left with a vague feeling that the treatment for cancer is morphia. This is largely an educational problem and underlies the purpose of this book.

Reference

Fowler, J. F. *Clin. Radiol.*, 1972, **23**, 257.

2

Physical Aspects

There are an ample number of excellent physics textbooks available. It is only necessary to remind the reader of a few of the more important points.

ENERGY

One aspect of physics concerns the study of different forms of energy (Table II). Although apparently quite different, these energy forms are often interchangeable.

TABLE II

Energy forms

Potential energy
Kinetic energy (including sound)
Electric energy
Chemical energy
Heat energy
Electromagnetic radiation
Nuclear energy

ELECTROMAGNETIC RADIATION

Electromagnetic radiation is a form of energy propagated by wave motion. The electromagnetic spectrum is shown in Figure 1. It ranges from radio waves of long wavelength ($\lambda = 3 \times 10^4$ m) and low frequency ($\nu = 10^4$ Hertz) to X-rays of short wavelength ($\lambda = 10^{-12}$ m) and high frequency ($\nu = 3 \times 10^{20}$ Hertz). In a vacuum electromagnetic waves travel at the velocity of light which is a constant, $C = 3 \times 10^8$ m/sec. The various wave forms are related by the formula $C = \nu\lambda$.

DUAL THEORY

Radiation has been presented above as a wave travelling through space. Alternatively it can be considered as a discontinuous stream of discrete

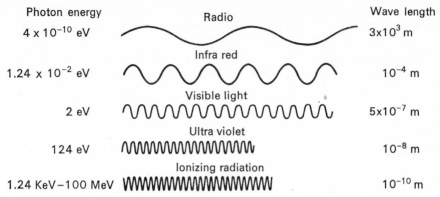

Figure 1 The electromagnetic spectrum

packets of energy or quanta — the photons. The size of each quantum is proportional to the frequency and is given by the formula:

$$E = h\nu$$

where E is the energy in electron volts, and h = Planck's constant.

IONIZING RADIATION

When the energy of photons exceeds a certain value, ionization occurs. High energy photons colliding with atoms overcome the electron binding energy of the outer atomic shells. Loosely bound electrons are removed from the shells leaving behind ionized atoms. These 'excited' atoms are chemically reactive, and are mainly responsible for radiobiological damage in living tissues. (See Chapter 3.)

ABSORPTION OR RADIATION

When a beam of ionizing radiation passes through matter, some of the radiation is scattered and some is absorbed. The relative amount of radiation emerging, $\frac{I}{I_0}$, depends on the photon energy of the radiation, the atomic number of the absorbing material, the thickness (t), and the density (ρ) of absorber used. Combining the absorber's properties into one characteristic (μ), for monochromatic radiation, the intensity (I) of the emergent beam is given by:

$$I = I_0 e^{\mu t}$$

where I_0 is the initial intensity and μ the absorption coefficient.

The factors involved in the attenuation of a radiation beam are:

1 **Scattering:** Both elastic and inelastic (Compton) scattering. This effect is mainly independent of atomic number.

2 **Photo-electric effect:** A photon disappears by interacting with a 'bound' electron. This effect dominates at low energies and high atomic numbers.

3 **Pair production:** A photon disappears and the energy is transformed into a positive and negative electron. This effect dominates at high energies and high atomic numbers. The reader is referred to the standard physics texts for more details on these important processes.

HALF-VALUE THICKNESS

The penetrating power or quality of an X-ray beam increases with the energy of the radiation. It is convenient to denote the penetrating power by the half-value thickness. This is the thickness of absorber necessary to reduce the intensity of a beam by 50 per cent. Half-value thicknesses are usually given in lead, copper or aluminium. In clinical practice, however, it is more meaningful to quote half-thicknesses in water.

INVERSE SQUARE LAW

The intensity of a beam of radiation decreases as the square of the distance (d) from a point source:

$$I \propto \frac{1}{d^2}.$$

The effect of the inverse square law is seen in the following situations:

1 The importance of considering source skin distance (SSD) in radiotherapy planning. For instance, the rapid fall-off in dose rate from superficial 'contact' X-ray therapy is due mainly to the short SSD rather than the low energy of the beam.

2 The large doses delivered by radium implants. The high intensity dosage is contained within a very small volume around the needles with minimal damage outside that zone.

3 The importance of distance in radiation protection.

RADIOACTIVITY

The nucleus of an atom is made up of protons and neutrons. For stable nuclei, these are present in about 50/50 ratio although neutrons tend to predominate in the heavier elements. Nuclei having a different proportion of neutrons and protons are unstable or radioactive and disintegrate, giving off various particles and energy (photons). Some unstable nuclei occur naturally (eg, radium); others are made artificially (eg, I^{131}). The decay of a radioactive isotope takes place exponentially as a function of time to a more stable form.

The time taken to decay to one half of any initial value is known as the half-life.

The activity of a radioactive source is measured in curies. A source is said to have an activity of one curie if $3 \cdot 7 \times 10^{10}$ disintegrations take place per second.

RADIATION MEASUREMENT

Radiation exposure is usually measured by the ionization it induces in air. The unit of X-ray quantity is the roentgen. The roentgen is defined as the amount of radiation, per cc of air at NTP, that produces one electrostatic unit of charge. This can be measured conveniently in an ionization chamber by measuring the passage of current across two charged electrodes. A more recent definition obviated the need for specifying NTP by defining the roentgen as follows:

$$1 \text{ roentgen} = 2 \cdot 58 \times 10^{-4} \text{ coulombs/kg air.}$$

Although the intensity of radiation from a source is measured in roentgens, measuring the radiation dose in roentgens is strictly speaking, incorrect. The dose is not determined by the number and energy of photons passing through a volume element during exposure, but by the amount of radiation that will be absorbed in different tissues. The unit of absorbed dose is the rad.

The absorbed dose in rads is the energy per unit mass actually imparted by the ionizing particles to the tissues within the volume element. One rad is equal to 100 ergs/g. If a dose of one rad is given to a cell, a portion of tissue or an organ, then irrespective of its chemical composition in the body, irrespective of its proximity to lead, bone or any other high atomic number material, and irrespective of the kind of radiation used, each gramme of irradiated tissue will have received an increase in energy of 100 ergs.

Unfortunately, the direct measurement of rads in a calorimeter is not a practical possibility because such large radiation doses are required to raise the temperature a measurable amount. In fact, the process of energy conversion is so efficient that the amount of electromagnetic energy necessary to kill a human being (1000 rads) would not produce a measurable temperature rise in a calorimeter. Indeed a dose of 100 000 rads only raises the temperature $0 \cdot 25$ degrees centigrade.

Thus, for practical purposes, we are forced to use the ionization rate in air as a means of measurement. However, it is possible to convert roentgens into rads, so long as the energy of the radiation and the atomic number of the tissue are known. For instance, one roentgen of conventional X-rays corresponds to an absorbed dose of $0 \cdot 86$ rads in air or $0 \cdot 93$ rads in water. In the megavoltage range the differential absorption in different tissues is disappearing (Figure 2) and the difference is even less important.

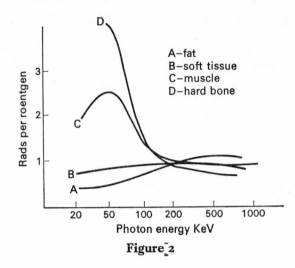

Figure 2

Other units which have been used are:

THE GRAM-RAD. The energy absorbed by a given volume of tissue is called the integral absorbed dose. It is measured in gram-rads.

$$1 \text{ g rad} = 100 \text{ ergs.}$$

It is desirable to keep the integral dose as low as possible since irradiation of large volumes of tissue produces inevitable side-effects.

THE REM (RAD EQUIVALENT MAN). The rem is equal to the dose of any ionization which when delivered to man is biologically equivalent to one rad of X-rays. It is intended to take account of the relative biological effectiveness (RBE) which is discussed later.

$$\text{Rem} = \text{Rad} \times \text{Quality Factor (QF)}$$

RADIATION SOURCES

Ionizing radiation can be obtained from X-ray machines, high energy accelerators, nuclear reactors or radioactive isotopes.

Conventional X-rays are generated in an X-ray tube. Electrons emitted from a hot filament impinge upon a tungsten target releasing X-rays at right angles. Energies of up to 300 kV can be attained this way.

The linear accelerator is one of the most popular high energy megavoltage machines in use today. Electrons from a gun are accelerated along a wave guide to velocities approaching that of light. A stable high output is attained at energies up to 35 MeV. The electrons can be extracted directly for treatment if required. Alternatively, the electrons may be directed at a target and emerge as megavoltage X-rays. Higher energy electrons may be obtained from betatrons. Further details are discussed in Chapter 23.

Artificial radioactive isotopes may be used as radiation sources. These are housed in teletherapy units with bulky treatment heads. The most widely used isotopes have been cobalt 60 and caesium 137. Large volume radiation sources are necessary, and these unfortunately give rise to penumbra at the edge of the treatment field. Although this can be trimmed, the sharp definition of the linear accelerator is not possible. Cobalt 60 has a higher specific activity and lower self absorption than caesium 137. But the shorter half-life of cobalt means that the source must be replaced every few years. A comparison of the physical properties of the two isotopes is given in Table III. Some caesium units have been designed with a short source skin distance. This combines the advantage of good quality radiation with rapid fall-off in dose rate below the skin surface.

DEPTH DOSE CURVES

When a beam of radiation is directed at a patient, the intensity usually decreases with the depth below the surface skin. The fall-off depends on the radiation quality, the field size and the SSD. The combined effects of these three factors can be measured in water and displayed as percentage depth dose curves (Figure 3).

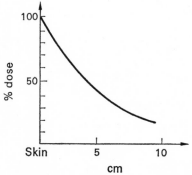

Figure 3   Depth dose curve

For the purpose of treatment planning it is better to use isodose curves. These add an extra dimension and show the extent of the penumbra at the edge of the treatment fields (Figure 4).

RADIOACTIVE ISOTOPES

A discussion of the numerous diagnostic and research applications of radioactive isotopes is beyond the scope of this book. The number of radioisotopes of value to the radiotherapist is more limited. Some of those with an established place in the armamentarium are given in Table III.

TABLE III

Radioactive isotopes

Radioactive isotopes	Radiation	Energy	Half-life	Comments
Phosphorus 32	Beta	1·17 MeV	14 days	Absorbed in tissues with a rapid turnover, eg, spleen and marrow. Used in polycythaemia
Gold 198	Gamma Beta	412 kV 0·96 MeV	2·7 days	Gold grains have largely replaced radon seeds. (HVT = 1/10" lead c.f. 1/2" lead for radon.) Also used in colloidal form in malignant effusions
Cobalt 60	Gamma	1·25 MeV	5·3 years	Specific activity = 400. HVT = 1/2" lead
Caesium 137	Gamma	0·66 MeV	33 years	Specific activity = 80. HVT = 1/4" lead
Iridium 192	Gamma	0·3 MeV to 0·612 MeV	74 days	Convenient for 'afterloading' implants
Strontium 90	Beta	0·546 MeV	28 years	Eye applicator. Sr^{90}/Yt^{90} in equilibrium are used for teletherapy

Yttrium 90	Beta	2·27 MeV	2·54 days	Rods for pituitary implants
Technetium 99	Gamma	140 kV	6 hours	Obtained from parent molybdenum 'cow'. Excellent for scanning because low energy allows good collimation and protection. 'Mistaken' for iodine biologically
Iodine 132	Gamma Gamma Gamma Beta	0·67 MeV 0·955 MeV 0·77 MeV 2·12 MeV	2·3 hours	See text
Iodine 131	Beta Gamma	0·81 keV 0·364 keV	8 days	See text
Iodine 125	Gamma Beta	35 kV 21 kV	60 days	See text
Iodine 124	Positrons	2·14 MeV	4·15 days	See text
Iodine 123	Gamma	159 kV	13 hours	See text
Californium 252	Neutrons Gamma	1 MeV (63%) 0·5–1 MeV (37%)	2·6 years	Suitable for interstitial and intracavitary therapy. The isotope has the advantage of higher LET than gamma emitters. Afterloading techniques are utilized since the personnel radiation hazard is 2·5 times greater than that for radium

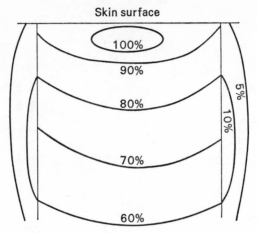

Figure 4   Isodose curve

Radioactive iodine 131 has been used for the diagnosis and treatment of thyroid disease over many years. The isotope has certain disadvantages. For instance, in large doses it has been known to cause pulmonary fibrosis. A number of other radio-isotopes of iodine are now available.

I^{132} gives a low dose to the thyroid compared with I^{131}. It is useful for quick uptake studies but is of no value in scanning.

I^{125} labelled compounds show good radiation stability and give resolution in autoradiography comparable to tritium. This isotope has limited application for *in vivo* tracer studies but can be used for protein-bound iodine estimation or urinary excretion tests. More recently, the low energy electrons from I^{124} have been used for therapeutic purposes. Most of the energy absorbed by the thyroid colloid is short range. Results are comparable to I^{131} therapy.

I^{124} emits positrons. These have a greater range than the beta particles from I^{131} and the isotope has been recommended for thyroid carcinoma where it gives more uniform irradiation. It is expensive.

I^{123} can only be produced in a cyclotron. Its short half-life makes it a safe isotope to use in pregnancy. It is also indicated when repeated scans are required or for thyroid investigations in children.

RADIATION PROTECTION

Ionizing radiation is dangerous: acute exposure leads to changes ranging from mild erythema of the skin to massive necrosis and death. Chronic exposure to low intensity radiation may induce malignant disease. Many early radiation workers were unaware of these dangers and developed epitheliomas of the skin. Others succumbed to leukaemia. Ionizing radiation also causes genetic damage with an increased mutation rate. In addition to these hazards, radiation is known to accelerate ageing. Exposure to small doses of X-rays over a long period of time increases the risk of premature death from myocardial infarction, bronchopneumonia and a number of other diseases. A study of life span among early radiologists showed that they died on an average 6 years earlier than other physicians. Happily, with present day safeguards this is no longer the case. (See also Chapter 4.)

Today routine blood counts for X-ray workers are mandatory. Radiation causes a pancytopenia. A fall in white cell count occurs shortly after exposure to moderate doses of radiation. Since red cells are relatively long-lived, anaemia is a late sign of damage. The platelet count also falls in the later stages. Very small amounts of radiation damage may be detected by chromosomal analysis of lymphocytes, but these studies are still in the experimental stage.

When the above changes are evident in the peripheral blood stream, the damage has already occurred. For this reason, radiation protection is mainly the responsibility of health physics departments.

TABLE IV

Relative hazards of radio-isotopes

Group	Radio-isotope
I	Ra^{226}
II	Sr^{90}; Rn^{222}
III	Co^{60}; I^{131}
IV	C^{14}; Na^{24}; P^{32}; Au^{198}

Most protection work is concerned with the dangers of external radiation but radioactive isotopes may be inhaled, ingested or absorbed through skin and orifices. A list of some toxic radio-isotopes is given in Table IV. The groups are arranged in decreasing order of hazard. Toxicity depends on a number of factors. For instance, although Carbon 14 has a long physical half-life, it is rapidly eliminated by the body and is a relatively safe substance to handle.

MAXIMUM PERMISSIBLE DOSE

Since the effects of ionizing radiation are cumulative, safe working conditions demand that the dose received should be as low as possible. There is probably no safe threshold dose below which radiation damage does not occur. However, mankind has evolved in the presence of background cosmic radiation. Hence it would seem reasonable if maximal permissible doses (MPD) were defined so that the risks involved were small compared with the ordinary hazards of life and industry.

For the purposes of protection, the dose limit set for radiation workers is higher than that set for the general population. This is because the inevitable long-term damage to the total genetic pool of distant generations will be 'diluted' if a relatively small number of people are involved.

The recommended MPD levels for the radiation worker are as follows:

Whole body	5 rem per year
Bone, thyroid, skin	30 rem per year
Extremities	75 rem per year

Fuller details are contained in the Recommendations of the International Commission on Radiological Protection (ICRP) published in 1966.

SI UNITS

The International Committee of Weights and Measures has developed a universal metric system — the International System of Units (SI). This system may be gradually introduced in radiotherapy over the next few years. One hundred rads would become one joule per kg and the unit of exposure would become one coulomb per kg. The curie was originally defined in terms of the disintegration of radium. A satisfactory SI unit to replace the curie has not yet been suggested.

References

Basic Radiation Protection Criteria, ICRP Report 39, 1971.

Gillespie, F. C., and Grieg, W. R. *Dose Distribution from I^{125}*, Brit. J. Radiol., 1970.

Johns, H. F., and Cunningham, J. R. *The Physics of Radiology*, Charles C. Thomas, 1971.

Meredith, W. J., and Massey, J. B. *Fundamental Physics of Radiology*, Williams & Wilkins, Baltimore, 1972.

3

Radiobiological Aspects

Physical Chemistry

Radiation has a direct and an indirect action on living cells: (1) direct energy absorption by cellular molecules results in broken chemical bonds; (2) most radiation damage is caused by indirect action. Ionizing radiation dissipates its energy through ion pairs with electron ejection in 10^{-13} seconds. These changes usually occur in water where H, OH and HO_2 radicals are produced, the exact amount of each depending on the amount of oxygen present. Many of these radicals recombine harmlessly to form water again. Others interact with nearby macromolecules causing bond breakage and an overall chemical change. This creates a biological system in which various 'foreign' chemicals have been produced and some vital constituents destroyed. Some of this damage occurs in the DNA molecule or possibly in the nuclear membrane, causing disruption of cellular function.

Cell Damage

The above changes hinder subsequent metabolism causing observable biological effects. Cell damage is difficult to measure precisely. Immediate cell death occurs only after enormous doses of radiation. Morphologically intact cells may persist after medium doses of X-rays, but such cells are not necessarily viable. Moreover, irradiated cells may divide several times before dying. Various end-points have been used to measure radiation damage. These include:

1   **Chromosome damage.** This is the most important cause of cell death but it usually cannot be observed until mitosis.
2   **Mutations.** These occur randomly and are an insensitive index of injury at low doses.
3   **Delay in division.**
4   **Loss of reproductive ability.** This is one of the most important measurements in radiation therapy.

Mammalian Cell Survival Curves

Puck and Marcus have made it possible to study the effects of radiation on mammalian cells *in vitro* rather than on plants and fruit flies. Single cells can be grown in clones on the surface of tissue culture dishes. The number of colonies observed following irradiation can then be counted and compared to controls.

Radiobiological results are often quoted in terms of the cell survival curve (Figure 5). This graph is obtained by plotting the fraction of a cell population which survives against radiation dose. The curve is almost exponential. The optimum mathematical point on an exponential curve is given by the formula $1/e = 0.37$. Thus the dose required to reduce the number of cells in a population to 37 per cent of the original number is called D37. This is a useful parameter for describing the survival curve.

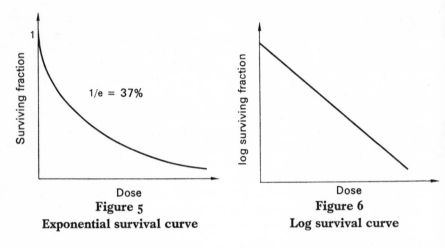

Figure 5   Figure 6
Exponential survival curve   **Log survival curve**

It is helpful visually to plot survival curves with the surviving fraction on a logarithmic scale (Figure 6). The exponential curve then becomes a straight line.

D37 is one index of radiosensitivity. For most cells its value lies between 80 and 200 rads with an average value of 130 rads. These values are lower than might be expected from the apparent radiosensitivities of parenchymal cells of various organs.

Extrapolation Number (N)

In practice, the logarithmic curve is not exactly a straight line. There is a small 'shoulder' to overcome before the curve is exponential (Figure 7). By extrapolation this shoulder can be measured on the vertical axis as N. N is called the extrapolation number and usually lies between 1.5 and 10 with an average value of 3. It measures a different parameter of radiosensitivity, threshold resistance.

Strictly speaking the slope of the exponential part of a Puck curve is given by D_0. D37 is not quite the same thing since it includes the shoulder of the curve. D_0 is more commonly used in the literature nowadays.

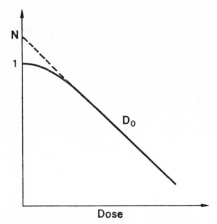

Figure 7   The shoulder and extrapolation number

Multitarget Law

On theoretical grounds one can postulate N targets in each cell. Each target must be hit once for total damage to occur. If less than N targets are hit, then sub-lethal injury ensues. Assuming this model, the cell survival curve is drawn as an exponential after an initial shoulder.

An alternative 'multihit' law has been proposed where each cell contains one target that must be hit N times. Both models are compatible with a mechanism of sub-lethal damage, when either the number of targets hit or the number of hits per target is below that required for lethal damage.

Recovery from Sub-Lethal Damage

When a given dose of radiation is divided into two increments, the biological effect is usually less than if the same amount of radiation had been delivered in a single dose. Partial recovery follows the first damaging event. The 'shoulder' is reproduced on the cell survival curve.

If F_1 represents the fraction surviving following single-dose irradiation, and F_2 the fraction surviving when the same dose has been given in two separate fractions, then F_2 is greater than F_1. $\dfrac{F_2}{F_1}$ is called the split-dose survival ratio. It measures cellular recovery following simple fractionation.

Following moderate doses of radiation, some recovery is of the sub-lethal variety and is thought to be due to biological repair. The remainder is by repopulation from undamaged cells.

The Cell Cycle

The cell cycle is illustrated in Figure 8. RNA and protein synthesis occur throughout interphase, but DNA synthesis occurs only during a part of interphase. It is preceded and followed by two gaps, G_1 and G_2. The cell then enters mitosis, dividing into two daughter cells. Mitosis is a very short period relative to the cell cycle. D_0 may vary by 50 per cent, depending at what point on the cell cycle irradiation takes place. The extrapolation number may vary even more than this.

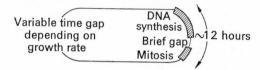

Figure 8   The cell cycle

The Oxygen Effect and OER

In anoxic conditions, repair following irradiation is by simple electron capture. In the presence of oxygen, the highly reactive radicals combine with oxygen and cause irreparable chemical damage. Therefore, for very small changes in oxygen tension, D_0 varies considerably. If a dose D is required to cause a fixed amount of damage in aerobic conditions, then mD is required to cause the same damage in anoxic conditions. m is known as the oxygen enhancement ratio (OER). It is about 2·5–3 for X-rays and gamma rays. A more accurate measurement of OER is derived from a comparison of cell survival curves rather than a comparison of single levels of damage.

LET

Ionizing radiation dissipates energy as it passes through tissue. This transfer of energy per micron of tissue is known as linear energy transfer (LET). LET is usually expressed in units of keV per micron. Some values of LET for different types of radiation are given in Table V. High LET means 'densely ionizing'; ie, more energy is dissipated per micron of track.

TABLE V

LET *values*

	Energy	**LET** (keV/μ)
Alpha particles	low energy	260
	5 MeV	95
Neutrons	slow, 2·5 MeV	20
	fast, 14 MeV	7
Protons	2 MeV	16
	10 MeV	4
X-rays	200 kV	0·4–36
Gamma rays	Cobalt 60	0·2–2
Electrons	1 MeV	0·25

RBE

Radiation becomes more efficient at high LET values. This is probably because each particle track is more damaged than those of electrons set going by X-rays. The relative biological effectiveness (RBE) measures this factor. It is defined as the ratio of doses of different radiations required to give the same biological effect. There is no single value of RBE for any pair of radiations, since the result depends on the parameter used to measure it. It also depends on the cell survival level chosen for these measurements. With high LET radiation, survival curves may be two or three times steeper than those obtained at low LET. High LET radiation has another advantage. The 'shoulder' on the cell survival curve becomes smaller, and extrapolation numbers approach unity. This is probably because the passage of a single high LET particle is sufficient to kill the cell, leaving no opportunity for recovery from sub-lethal injury. At lower LETs, multiple tracks arriving at different times allow radicals to recombine harmlessly into water; high LET single track damage allows no time for this inter-current repair.

Relationship between LET and OER

Oxygen is less effective in enhancing damage at high LETs. This may be because free oxygen is formed in the tracks of heavily ionizing particles. Thus, fast neutrons have an OER which is less than that found with X-rays by a factor of $1 \cdot 6$.

Radiosensitizing Agents

The search for radiosensitizing drugs has been going on for 50 years. A true radiosensitizer should act at a non-toxic dose level. So far oxygen is the only agent that fulfils this criterion *in vivo*, although some of the halogenated pyrimidines have been shown to work *in vitro*.

Non-metabolizing sensitizers are being investigated. These act like oxygen on hypoxic cells but diffuse further into the tumour without being metabolized en route. NDPP has been the most successful but its pharmacology and toxicity have not yet been tested.

A number of cytotoxic and other drugs have been used empirically with variable results. These include alkylating agents, actinomycin D, ethylhydrazide of podophyllic acid and porphyrins. However at toxic dose levels, simple additive effects cannot be excluded, and such drugs cannot be considered radiosensitizers.

Timed doses of methotrexate and hydroxyurea have been used to induce synchrony in cell division and hopefully exploit the most radiosensitive phase of the cell cycle. Results have not yet been fully assessed, but the drugs also affect normal tissues and it may be difficult to achieve differential destruction.

Radioprotective Agents

Normal tissues may be partly protected from radiation by inducing anoxia. This can be produced using a tourniquet on the limb or by hypothermia. Local anoxia may be enhanced by vasoconstrictor and related compounds such as adrenaline, histamine or serotonin.

Direct radioprotective drugs have been sought. Cysteine and cysteamine have been used extensively in animal experiments but are somewhat toxic. Aminothiol compounds have also been studied. One of these, thiouracil, is known to reduce the effectiveness of radio-iodine therapy. It was hoped to use some of these products to develop protective creams and ointments for the skin, intestinal tract and vagina. So far results have been disappointing. However the very high radioresistance of certain plants and fungi suggests that effective radioprotective agents may yet be found.

FRACTIONATION

In the early days of radiotherapy, fractionation developed along empirical lines. It is only recently that an attempt has been made to rationalize fractionation patterns. The clinical advantages of fractionation are apparent: for instance, it is possible to cure cancer of the lip with a single dose of about 2100 rads. If the same radical dose were given to a large abdominal tumour in a single treatment, the side-effects would be intolerable. Thus when large volumes of tissue are irradiated, treatment must be fractionated over a period of time. An additional advantage of fractionation is that the patient's response to treatment may be observed. If a brisk initial reaction occurs, it is possible to stop treatment prematurely and avoid excessive damage.

It is more difficult to sustain the argument that repeated daily fractionation spares normal tissue at the expense of tumour tissue. Radiobiological experiments have shown that with conventionally fractionated radiation at a cellular level, sub-lethal injuries are repaired and the 'shoulder' reduplicated with each daily fraction. This accounts for the increased total dose necessary with fractionation. This daily duplication of the 'shoulder' is not an efficient use of energy as far as cell suppression is concerned.

At a tissue level it is difficult to interpret findings. Most radiobiologists now believe that as the tumour shrinks, fractionation allows better oxygenation in the latter stages of treatment. Others claim that the dose should be increased towards the end of treatment because arteriolar narrowing and thrombosis reduce oxygenation. The time factors for these changes are not known accurately, but reduced oxygenation due to fibrosis probably only becomes important after several months.

Complicated dynamic fractionation patterns have been proposed in an attempt to match the dose to the individual tumour. However, there is no evidence that this is of any value.

NSD

The biological effect of a dose of radiation depends not only on the time taken to deliver the dose but also on the number of treatments employed. The relationship between dose, time and fractionation can be put in empirical mathematical terms using the Ellis formula. The formula allows comparisons of treatment plans with widely different fractionation patterns by reducing the overall dose given during a course of treatment to a nominal standard dose (NSD) measured in rets. It states that:

$$D = NSD \times N^{0.24} \times T^{0.11}$$

where D is the total dose delivered, N is the number of fractions and T the overall treatment time measured in days. The formula indicates that the number of fractions is a more dominant factor than the elapsed time in days.

In the United Kingdom, a Fractionation Working Party has presented some preliminary data on different fractionation patterns. No meaningful analysis can yet be made but it seems clear that there is little difference in changing from five fractions per week to three fractions per week, so long as the overall total dose is reduced by 10 to 15 per cent. Thus it appears that, although it may be some time before we can fully exploit the radiobiological possibilities of fractionation, it may soon be possible to simplify current clinical regimens without loss of effectiveness.

The subject of fractionation is also discussed in Chapter 5.

References

Alper, T. *Modern Trends in Radiotherapy*, ed. Deely and Wood, 1967, **1**, 1.

Ellis, F. *Dose, Time and Fractionation: A Clinical Hypothesis*, Clin. Radiol., 1968, **20**, 1.

Fowler, J. F. *Current Aspects of Radiobiology as applied to Radiotherapy*, Clin. Radiol., 1972, **23**, 257.

Little, J. B. *Cellular Effects of Ionizing Radiation*, New Eng. J. Med., 1968, **278**, 308.

4

Radiation Pathology

The previous section discussed the effects of ionizing radiation on mammalian cells. These effects are now considered in relation to individual tissues, then to the whole body, and finally in relation to malignant cells.

Skin

Radiation damage to the skin is often the limiting factor in radiotherapy. The dose determines the amount of damage. Individual variation is considerable depending on race, sex, age and other factors. For instance, pigmented races can tolerate slightly higher doses than white races. The average observed changes following single exposures of X-ray therapy are listed below:

500 rads	Temporary epilation lasting one month.
1000 rads	Erythema, temporary epilation, pigmentation.
1500 rads	Erythema, temporary epilation, pigmentation, dry desquamation.
2000 rads and above	Erythema, permanent epilation, moist desquamation. This may lead to healing with telangiectasia. Higher doses cause necrosis.

The histological changes in the epidermis and dermis resemble an inflammatory reaction with subsequent repair and regeneration. There are also pigmentary changes due to extravasation of iron and melanocyte migration.

Permanent suppression of the cutaneous appendages is achieved with the following single dosages:

Sebaceous glands	1250 rads
Hair follicles	1750 rads
Sweat glands	2250 rads

The changes seen depend on dose fractionation. Following massive single doses, acute radionecrosis of skin develops rapidly without a latent period. On the other hand, following small protracted doses, chronic radiation dermatitis with dry cracked skin, atrophic nail changes and indolent ulceration may not occur for many years.

Lungs

Radiation damage to the lungs may occasionally occur following treatment of such conditions as breast cancer or Hodgkin's disease. When the dose to the entire lung exceeds 2500 rads in 3 weeks the following changes are seen:

1   Lymph follicles degenerate with hyperaemia of the bronchial mucosa.
2   One month latent period.
3   Acute inflammatory reaction of alveoli, followed by degeneration of bronchial epithelium.
4   Regeneration leading to fibrosis. This process takes about 6 months.

Clinically the patient may have symptoms of pneumonitis during the inflammatory phase. Later, in the fibrotic phase, he may develop cough, haemoptysis and dyspnoea. Patients with normal pulmonary function, however, can tolerate up to 25 per cent destruction of pulmonary volume without difficulty.

The late radiographic changes are as follows:

1   Fibrosis with shrinkage pulling the trachea out of midline.
2   Lung opacity.
3   Radiation rib fractures ('tooth-edge' breaks with no bone lysis).
4   Pleural reaction.

Urinary System

The kidneys are at risk during any form of abdominal irradiation as in the treatment of seminoma. For this reason, it is essential to shield renal tissue where possible. Radiation nephritis often develops when the dose exceeds 2000 rads in 5 weeks. At first no changes are observed. After a latent interval, an inflammatory infiltrate of lymphocytes and plasma cells invades the irradiated area. Parenchymal cells are swollen, and there is oedema of the interstitial tissue. Vascular damage with end-arteritis is also noted. Eventually fibrotic changes supervene.

Clinically the patient with radiation nephritis presents with anaemia, hypertension and albuminuria 6 months after irradiation. A few cases present with a frank nephrotic syndrome. Most cases eventually die in renal failure. Fortunately, this is a rare occurrence today.

The bladder tolerates up to 5000 rads in 5 weeks. Radiation cystitis is transient at these dose levels. Higher doses may lead to ulceration and eventual shrinkage with contracted bladder.

Central Nervous System

Neurological tissue is relatively radioresistant. This may be because central nervous tissue cells are non-dividing. Nevertheless electrical conduction studies of nervous tissue in frogs have shown functional damage after doses as low as 300 rads. Histologically, the changes vary from mild gliosis to necrosis depending on the dose. These effects may be largely due to indirect vascular damage rather than nervous tissue damage.

In clinical practice the human brain will tolerate doses up to 4000 rads in 4 weeks. Smaller volumes of tissue may be taken to higher doses.

In the treatment of neck lesions such as thyroid carcinoma, there is a danger of inducing radiation myelitis after a latent period of up to one year. This hazard was originally reported by Boden in 1948. It was noted that the risk increases with the length of cord irradiated. Permanent damage has been reported when the dose to a 20 cm length of cord exceeded 1200 rads single or 3000 rads in 3 weeks. Neurological changes vary between slight sensory disturbance to paraplegia with incontinence.

Intestinal Tract

Intestinal damage may occur following abdominal irradiation as in the treatment of ovarian carcinoma. Cells lining the small gut divide rapidly and show damage after doses as low as 200 rads. In clinical practice, however, fractionated doses up to 3000 rads may be well tolerated. Microscopically, the first changes noted in the epithelium are large swollen misshapen cells. Cell debris then collects in the crypts of Lieberkuhn. Later on, vascular damage may lead to ischaemic changes.

In the acute phase patients may complain of nausea, vomiting, abdominal pain, diarrhoea and tenesmus. Paralytic ileus may develop. In the late stages, following indiscriminate irradiation, patients may develop fistulae or strictures. Malabsorption syndrome and protein-losing gastro-enteropathy have also been described.

Eyes

The eye is sometimes irradiated in the treatment of conditions such as carcinoma of the maxillary antrum. The lens is the most sensitive part of the eye. Lenticular opacities have been seen following doses as low as 200 rads single or 400 rads in 4 weeks. Doses above 1150 rads will cause cataracts in all patients. Radiation cataracts may take years to develop, however. The first change noted is a small dot at the posterior pole of the lens. This enlarges, and vacuoles and granules appear round the opacity, creating a 'doughnut' appearance. This is followed by yellow hue opacities with a bivalve configuration in the pupillary area. Thereafter the changes are indistinguishable from other cataracts.

Ulcerating conjunctivitis is one of the earliest signs of radiation damage. A dose of over 5500 rads in 3 weeks will destroy the eye completely.

Bone

In the treatment of childhood malignancy, it is important to appreciate that the growing epiphyses are extremely radiosensitive. Early changes are seen when the dose exceeds 500 rads in 1 week. Larger doses lead to growth stunting and arrest. Careful alignment of treatment fields helps reduce this danger.

In the adult, medium doses of X-rays are well tolerated, but larger doses lead to limb deformity and osteonecrosis with sequestra formation.

Bone marrow suppression has already been discussed.

Gonads

These are the most radiosensitive organs. Up to 300 rads may be tolerated without loss of fertility, although long-term genetic damage may occur with lower doses. On the other hand, many patients have had normal children following higher doses. Permanent sterility is usually induced when the dose exceeds 1200 rads in 4 days to the ovaries. It is important to remember that an artificial menopause will be induced in most young women receiving pelvic irradiation.

WHOLE BODY RADIATION INJURY

Low dose exposure to whole body radiation over a long period of time has already been discussed. Such exposure leads to an increased risk of malignant disease, particularly leukaemia and to a general increase in ageing of all tissues.

Following acute high dose accidental radiation exposure, a variable time elapses before the onset of symptoms. The subsequent radiation syndrome is divided into three stages depending on the dose received.

The haematological syndrome occurs at single doses above 200 rads. All the elements in the bone marrow are depressed as shown in Figure 9. The lymphocytes are the first cells affected, and the total white cell count is usually depressed inside 48 hours. Erythrocytes have a normal life span of about 140 days, and the red cell count only begins to fall 1 week after exposure.

The gastro-intestinal syndrome occurs at single doses above 700 rads, but there is considerable overlap with the haematological syndrome. Anorexia and nausea may occur inside a few hours. At higher doses this may progress to vomiting and intestinal obstruction. Diarrhoea occurring inside 48 hours suggests that very high doses have been received, and the outcome is often fatal.

The central nervous system syndrome occurs at single doses above 2000 rads. A constellation of symptoms and signs are seen ranging from headache and papilloedema to convulsions with coma. The syndrome is always fatal. In fact, no one has yet survived single whole body doses above 1000 rads.

The management of the patient depends on the dose received. This may

B

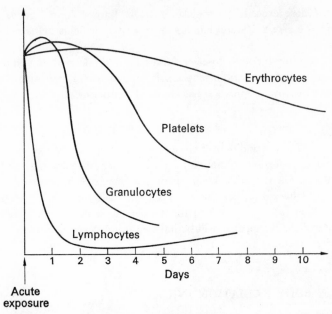

Figure 9   Blood picture following radiation exposure

be difficult to determine but the time gap before the onset of symptoms enables one to take the following preliminary therapeutic steps:

1   Treat associated burns and trauma.
2   Remove radioactive contamination.
3   Estimate the physical dose received.
4   Blood sampling for radiochemical analysis.
5   Neutrons may induce radioactivity. This should be checked on a whole body counter.

The clinical features may be helpful. Nausea, vomiting, diarrhoea, pallor, anxiety, lassitude or pyrexia during the first 12 hours indicate a grave prognosis and a dose in excess of 500 rads. Erythema developing within a few hours can also be serious, but may sometimes represent only superficial beta injury. Epilation during the first two weeks indicates that the skin dose exceeded 300 rads.

Following a fatal exposure, treatment should be limited to symptomatic measures giving fluid and electrolyte replacement together with sedation. For small exposures below 450 rads, however, bed rest and symptomatic measures may suffice.

Sub-lethal injury (less than 900 rads) should be dealt with as follows:

1   Bed rest.
2   Barrier nursing with antibiotic therapy.

3 Control bleeding:
   a Whole blood transfusion.
   b If petechia appear give large amounts of fresh concentrated platelets.
   c Bone marrow graft at the end of the first week. If the white cell count is low and the patient's condition is deteriorating, a leukocyte infusion may be given.
4 Gastro-intestinal damage with obstruction may require surgery in the third week.

RADIOSENSITIVITY

Bergonie and Tribondeau (1906) studied the effects of radiation on rat testes. They noted that radiosensitivity depends on the reproductive activity of the cell and is inversely proportional to the degree of differentiation. Well-differentiated slow-growing cells (eg, nerve and muscle cells) are radioresistant, whereas rapidly growing poorly differentiated cells (eg, germinal cells of ovary) are radiosensitive.

A corollary of this is Ellinger's law. This states that the radiosensitivity of a tumour reflects the radiosensitivity of the tissue it arises from (Table VI).

TABLE VI

Tissue radiosensitivity

Radiosensitivity	Tissues	Neoplasms
High	Embryonic Gonads Lymphoid	Wilm's tumour Seminoma Hodgkin's disease
Medium	Epithelial Glandular	Epidermoid carcinoma Adenocarcinoma
Low	Muscle tissue Fibrous tissue	Leiomyosarcoma Fibrosarcoma

Thus seminoma and dysgerminoma arising from the reproductive organs are extremely radiosensitive. Fibrosarcoma arising from fibrous tissue is relatively radioresistant.

It is often stated that radiosensitive tumours are not necessarily radio-curable. This is because these tumours may metastasize before treatment can be given. In clinical practice, radiosensitivity is defined as tumour regression with no local recurrence. It is, in fact, local radiocurability in the treated zone. It has nothing to do with the speed of tumour regression, although the two often parallel each other. The speed of tumour regression depends mainly on the rate of removal of dead cells from the treated zone.

Radiobiological experiments consistently show that most cells are about equally radiosensitive. As mentioned earlier, cell damage may not be seen until the subsequent mitosis, and this may not be due for some time. Moreover, damaged cells may mitose a few times before dying. Thus it is loss of reproductive activity and not immediate cell death that is important clinically. It is worth noting that post-irradiation biopsy specimens may show morphologically intact cells histologically. This does not necessarily imply that such cells are viable.

Formerly, X-ray therapy was based on the theory that rapidly dividing tumour cells were more sensitive than normal cells. The analogy was usually made that it is easier to trip up a man who is running than one who is walking. However, radiobiological experiments have now shown that, if anything, proliferating normal cells are more sensitive than many tumour cells. Hence today the Law of Bergonie and Tribondeau must be explained in terms of turnover rate or doubling-time of the cell population, and not as inherent differences in cellular radiosensitivity.

Notwithstanding the above remarks, most clinicians still feel that there are a number of tumours, such as malignant melanoma, whose radiosensitivity cannot yet be explained entirely in radiobiological terms. Other factors, possibly hormonal and immunological, may be important. These can interact with radiochemical changes to produce the final result.

Lastly, it should be noted that this discussion is limited to mammalian cells. Other forms of life have quite different levels of radiosensitivity. Indeed certain insects, plants and fungi can withstand enormous doses of ionizing radiation.

References

Boden, G. *Radiation Myelitis of the cervical spinal cord*, Brit. J. Radiol., 1948, **21**, 464.
Boden, G. *Radiation Myelitis of the brain stem*, Clin. Radiol., 1950, **2**, 79.
Paterson, R. *Renal Damage from Radiation*, Clin. Radiol., 1951, **3**, 270.
Rubin, P., and Casarett, G. *Clinical Radiation Pathology*, Saunders, Philadelphia, 1968.

5

Therapeutic Aspects

Evaluation

The first step in therapy is to assess the nature and extent of the disease. The site, stage, grade and length of history of the condition are all determined. At the same time, the patient's symptoms are considered since the main object of treatment may be simply to relieve discomfort. It is also important to know whether the patient is fit enough to undergo radical treatment. Age and general condition are noted. The presence of anaemia and coexistent disease such as infection, diabetes and arteriosclerosis are relevant.

Radical or Palliative

Perhaps the most important decision to reach before starting treatment is whether the disease is potentially curable or incurable.

General measures

These may involve bed rest, sedation, diet, blood transfusion and antibiotic therapy.

Psychological factors are particularly important in patients suffering from malignant disease. Most patients referred for radiation therapy know they have cancer; sometimes they have been told, more often they have guessed. The question of how frank the physician should be is controversial. It depends partly on the prognosis, but it is often as cruel to be evasive as it is to be brutally frank. The responsibility does not end with the physician. All those who come in contact with cancer patients in varying degrees should endeavour to use a combination of tact and understanding coupled with reassurance.

Specific Treatment

The treatment of choice at each anatomical site is discussed in the appropriate chapter. Each case must be considered on its merits. In some instances a combination of surgery, radiotherapy and chemotherapy is best.

TREATMENT TECHNIQUES

External Radiation

This is usually satisfactory for most radiotherapeutic situations. Superficial lesions can be treated with medium or low voltage X-rays but deeper lesions require supervoltage X-ray therapy. Supervoltage radiation has the following advantages over medium or orthovoltage radiation:

1. Better penetration of tissues.
2. Skin sparing.
3. Homogeneous absorption in bone and soft tissue.
4. Smaller integral dose.

Occasionally, megavoltage therapy is used to treat deep-seated lesions that extend on to the skin surface. In these cases the skin is covered with a tissue equivalent material such as wax or bolus to allow maximum build-up of dose on the surface of the treated area.

A single radiation field is satisfactory for some cases but a midline tumour is often better treated through a pair of parallel opposed fields (Figure 10). Multiple field therapy may be indicated where added skin protection is required (Figure 11). Rotation therapy is an extension of this

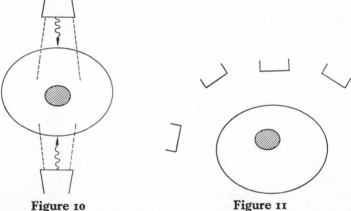

Figure 10
Parallel opposed fields

Figure 11
Multiple field therapy

concept (Figure 12). In rotation therapy the machine usually rotates around the patient although the converse is also possible. When the treatment plan calls for two fields directed at right angles to each other, as in carcinoma of the maxillary antrum, the use of wedge filters eliminates 'hot-spots' where adjacent field margins abut (Figure 13).

It is important to treat all the radiation portals at each treatment session. The practice of treating alternate fields on alternate days, which is used to save time in some busy understaffed centres, produces uneven biological dose patterns.

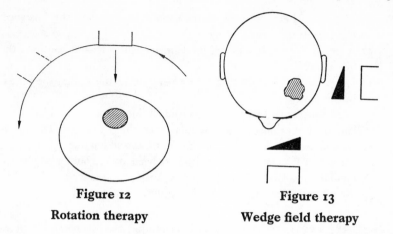

Figure 12

Rotation therapy

Figure 13

Wedge field therapy

Radium

This naturally occurring radioactive isotope has a half-life of 1600 years. It decays to radon gas and in the process emits good quality gamma rays. The dose rate from 1 mg radium filtered through 0·5 mm platinum at 1 cm distance is equal to 8·25 r/hr in air.

The use of radium enables enormous doses of radiation to be delivered to the tumour *in situ*. At the same time the rapid fall-off in dose rate provides maximum protection to surrounding normal tissue. Radium is used in the following situations:

1. INTRACAVITARY INSERTIONS. Intracavitary radium involves placing radium in a body cavity for the purpose of treating malignant disease in or around that cavity. The technique is mostly used today in the treatment of gynaecological cancer. The rules governing radium distribution in the female pelvis are discussed in the relevant sections of Chapter 17 and in the standard radium textbooks.

2. MOULDS. Radium mould treatments are mainly used for treatment of certain skin cancers, particularly those overlying cartilage. The technique is also used occasionally in oral cancer. Radium is mounted on applicators overlying the treatment zone. The aim is to deliver a certain dose to the skin surface at a fixed distance from the plane of the radium. Distribution rules have been formulated which produce a homogeneous field of radiation over the involved area. A few elementary rules are given below:

1   Moulds should be considered as planar if the curvature is less than that of a hemisphere.
2   Circles are the ideal shape.
3   The aim should be to use as many radioactive foci as possible, with an absolute minimum of six.

4 The space between each source should be less than the 'distance' from the treated surface.

5 A single circle will suffice if its diameter is less than three times the 'distance'.

6 Larger circles require that 3 to 5 per cent of the radium be placed in the centre.

7 With squares and rectangles, additional lines should be added if the length of the longer side exceeds twice the 'distance'. The linear radium density should be 50 per cent for the added line.

8 More detailed mathematical rules have been worked out for 'sandwich' moulds, line sources and cylinders. Again, the reader is referred to the references at the end of this chapter.

3. INTERSTITIAL IMPLANTS. In this technique the radioactive sources are implanted directly into the cancerous tissue, usually in the form of radium needles. There is, however, an important difference between interstitial radium therapy and superficial radium mould therapy. In mould therapy it is possible to obtain dose homogeneity, whereas in interstitial therapy there is an intensely high, though localized, zone of irradiation immediately around each implanted needle or seed. For most situations this is unimportant; indeed it may even be advantageous. Interstitial therapy is ideally suited for anatomical situations where the tumour is well localized in the tissues, such as cancer of the anterior part of the tongue. Small lesions up to 0·5 cm diameter may be treated by a single plane of radium needles. Larger tumours require two or more planes of needles. Reference tables are available quoting mg hr/1000 r at different distances from the needles.

The following distribution rules apply for simple cases:

1 Radium needles and radon seeds should not be placed more than 1 cm apart.

2 For areas under 25 sq. cm, two-thirds of the radium should be distributed around the periphery and one-third over the remaining area.

3 Ten per cent should be deducted from the area if one end of the implant is left open or 'uncrossed'.

Additional radium distribution rules have been published for more complex volume arrangements, such as a cylinder (see references).

Post-operative Radium Care

The procedure should be explained to patients before anaesthesia. Often patients try to remove the implant on awakening. Close observation for respiratory obstruction should be kept for 24 hours. It is important to get patients ambulant quickly and avoid chest infection. Nutrition should be maintained with glucose drinks since swallowing is difficult. A feeder cup with a rubber spout is useful. Smoking should be prohibited. The mouth must be rinsed frequently with a bland solution, such as sodium bicarbonate — 1 tsp to 1 pint of warm water. The nursing staff should also be instructed to ensure that radium needles are not dislodged and that radium moulds remain in a fixed position.

Radon and Gold Seeds

Radon is a gamma emitter with a half-life of 3·8 days. Because of the short half-life, interstitial radon seed implants can be left permanently in the tissues. Since it is not possible to remove the seeds, however, it is necessary to plan the treatment beforehand as carefully as possible. But occasionally the end-result may be somewhat different from the original plan, and this makes it difficult to obtain accurate dosimetry. For this reason, such treatment is usually combined with a course of external radiotherapy. This reduces any overall error but still permits adequate delivery of an intense zone of radiation to small localized tumour volumes.

The distribution rules for radon seeds follow those for radium. Each millicurie of radon is equivalent to 133·3 mg hours of radium. Dosimetry tables are available, quoting the average dose throughout the treated volume.

In the United Kingdom radon has been replaced by radioactive gold 198 seeds. This isotope has a half-life of 2·7 days. It is simpler to handle, and the lower half-life thickness makes it less hazardous to patients and staff.

Radioactive Isotopes

A number of radioactive isotopes have been used extensively in radio-therapeutic practice. Mention has already been made of the use of cobalt 60 and caesium 137 as gamma sources for external teletherapy. Less penetrating radiation may be obtained for treatment of superficial lesions from beta sources such as strontium 90. Radioactive iridium and caesium have also been used in place of radium and radon in interstitial and intracavitary work. Many of these substances are safer to handle and are suitable for afterloading. This technique, along with electron therapy, is discussed in Chapter 23.

Two other radio-isotopes have been used for their therapeutic potential. These are radiophosphorus in polycythaemia and radio-iodine in thyroid disease.

TREATMENT PLANNING

Meticulous attention to detail is rewarded in radiotherapy. It has been shown that dose variations of the order of 5 per cent can significantly influence survival. The various steps in accurate treatment planning are outlined below.

Localization

Precise localization of the tumour should be obtained where possible. Occasionally the surgeon may be able to outline the margins of the lesion with metal clips at the time of operation. Various radiographic techniques may also be used. These include lateral soft tissue views of the neck, tomograms, barium studies, cystograms and so on. These X-rays are usually taken with overlying metal skin markers.

Isodose Construction

An anatomical contour of the patient is made and the position of the tumour marked as accurately as possible. Isodose curves are then constructed and an optimum treatment plan designed. The portals of entry of the radiation fields are arranged to avoid vital structures such as the lens of the eye, rectum or spinal cord. The computer is being used more and more for this purpose. It can carry out dull repetitive tasks in a rapid manner, and the additional speed means that the therapist can now choose from a wide selection of treatment plans.

Beam Direction

Accurate beam direction is as important as localization. In attempting to correct to the nearest decimal point for all the variables, the therapist must not lose sight of the primary objective: that the beam be directed precisely at the target. Otherwise measurements of beam energy, filtration, LET dose, output, RBE, port size, distance, etc become merely academic exercises.

Several techniques are commonly used to ensure that the beam is pointing at the tumour. These include light-centring beams, back-pointers, a pin-and-arc device, and more recently, laser beams.

A beam direction shell may also be made. This involves making an **impression** of the anatomical contour using a substance such as Plaster-of-Paris bandage. A **model** is then constructed by pouring fluid Plaster-of-Paris into this impression. A rigid **applicator shell** is then constructed by moulding plastic material on to this model. The applicator shell has the advantage that the patient can be set in precisely the same position each day throughout treatment.

X-ray simulators are being used more frequently in radiotherapy departments. These machines simulate therapy in a mock-up room prior to the actual delivery of treatment. The alignment of the portals can thus be checked with a diagnostic quality film. Additionally this has the advantage of saving considerable setting-up time on the treatment unit, which can be devoted to other patients.

It is sometimes possible to take X-ray films with the megavoltage rays from the treatment unit. These verification films are often of poor quality but they can be helpful, especially in the pelvis, where there are no reliable skin landmarks.

MOVING STRIP THERAPY

Large doses of abdominal radiation are poorly tolerated. Thus, such treatment has to be given slowly over a period of several weeks, rendering it biologically less effective. One way of overcoming this is to split the area into smaller regions and treat each separately. However, gaps or overlapping may occur at the margins. For this reason moving strip therapy was devised. The abdomen is divided into a series of anterior and posterior horizontal strips 2·5 cm wide (Figure 14). The lowest strip is treated on the first day; then strips one and

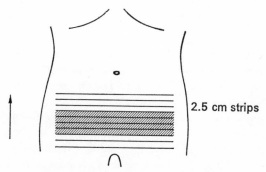

Figure 14   Moving strip therapy

two are treated on the second day; then strips one, two and three; and finally strips one to four. The four strips are then moved up the abdomen each day in steps of 2·5 cm. Care is taken to avoid vital structures such as the kidneys. Although the overall treatment still takes several weeks to deliver, the technique enables one to deliver an effective tumour dose of 3000 rads in 10 days to each strip.

Moving strip therapy assumes that the abdominal contents are fixed. This, of course, is not the case, and there may be overdosage or underdosage to loops of bowel and other mobile structures. Malignant cells in ascitic fluid may also move in and out of the X-ray beam.

DOSIMETRY

In prescribing treatment, the aim is to deliver a lethal dose to the tumour with minimum damage to the surrounding normal tissues.

The concept of fractionation has already been discussed, and it was noted that where large volumes of tissues are irradiated it is necessary to protract the treatment over an extended period of time. Over the years, empirical dose schedules have been obtained for different treatment situations. A selection is shown in Table VII. A glance at this emphasizes the importance of the treatment volume. This has led to the radiotherapeutic aphorism, 'large volume, small dose; small volume, large dose'. Thus care must be

TABLE VII

Fractionation patterns (5 treatments per week)

	Small fields (About 5 × 5 cm)	**Medium fields** (About 10 × 10 cm)	**Large fields** (Over 15 × 15 cm)
Single	2100 rads	1500 rads	500–1000 rads
1 week	3400 rads	2750 rads	1500 rads
2 weeks	4000 rads	3500 rads	2500 rads
3 weeks	5000 rads	4500 rads	3000 rads
4 weeks	5500 rads	5000 rads	4000 rads
5 weeks	6000 rads	5500 rads	4500 rads
6 weeks	7000 rads	6000 rads	5000 rads

taken to keep the volume as small as possible, compatible with covering a reasonable margin around the tumour. The volume factor has been analysed recently by the author in Table VIII. The inverse relationship is shown graphically in Figure 15.

The prescribed dose also depends on the radiosensitivity of the lesion. Whereas follicular lymphoma may respond to a dose of about 2000 rads in 2 weeks, epidermoid carcinoma of the mouth requires a dose of over 5000 rads in 4 weeks. The appropriate dose for each tumour is discussed in the relevant section.

TABLE VIII

Variation of dose with volume

	Dose (rets)	Volume (cm³)
Pituitary (protons)	4000	1
Superficial X-rays	3000	15
Radium	2500	150
Larynx	1900	350
Standard therapy	1800	1000
Total pelvis	1550	4500
Total abdomen	1320	13 000
Whole body	1000	70 000

There are five occasions when the dose should be reduced:

1 Old age. A reduction of 10 per cent.
2 Children. A reduction of 10 to 30 per cent.
3 Palliation. A reduction of up to 30 per cent.
4 Non-malignant disease. The dose is usually well below 50 per cent of a radical dose. (See individual condition.)
5 Pre-operative irradiation. A reduction of 20 to 30 per cent.

Split course therapy has been recommended in certain clinical situations. This consists in dividing a course of therapy into two separate phases with

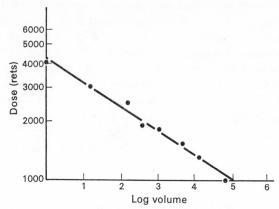

Figure 15   Dose volume relationship

a gap of up to 4 weeks between the first and second phase. The overall dose is somewhat higher than that delivered by orthodox fractionation. But several advantages have been claimed:

1 Treatment is better tolerated, especially in frail elderly patients.
2 The extended interval allows occult metastases time to manifest themselves and may spare such patients the possible morbidity associated with more radical therapy.
3 The treatment gap may allow better oxygenization of tissues and increased radiosensitivity during the latter part of therapy.
4 Tumour shrinkage following the gap enables one to irradiate smaller volumes during the latter part of treatment.

RADIATION AND SURGERY

A combination of radiation and surgery often produces the best result for the patient. This implies that the surgeon and the radiotherapist should be aware of what each can achieve, both individually and collectively. There is no substitute for close liaison between the two specialties. Sometimes surgery is recommended for the primary tumour with radiotherapy to the lymph node drainage areas. Sometimes the reverse is recommended with radiation to the primary and surgery to the lymph nodes. More often the question is simply one of pre-operative or post-operative radiation. Generally speaking, if combined therapy is being considered, it is preferable to give the radiation prior to surgery. This is alleged to reduce dissemination of disease at the time of surgery. But there are exceptions to this rule. For instance, the diagnosis and extent of disease may sometimes only be obtained at the time of surgery. Moreover it is self-evident that the surgical findings may completely alter the subsequent management of the case, eg, liver metastases.

It has already been mentioned that the pre-operative radiation dose should be kept below a radical therapeutic dose level. In addition to this, a delay of 6 weeks is recommended as the ideal gap between radiation and surgery. Immediately following radiation an inflammatory reaction sets in which begins to subside after 1 month. This delays healing. After several months radiation fibrosis develops, and subsequent surgery becomes extremely difficult. It is occasionally possible to operate on patients who have had a full radical course of radiotherapy. But this is usually only recommended where small volumes of tissue have been irradiated. In such cases an adequate margin of normal tissue around the involved area is essential for subsequent healing and repair.

PALLIATIVE RADIOTHERAPY

One of the most important contributions of radiotherapy is the palliative control of metastatic disease. Today such treatment should be closely co-ordinated with the chemotherapeutic management of the case. When localized symptoms develop, radiotherapy often provides the most rapid means of relief. Specific forms of palliative treatment are mentioned under the relevant anatomical sections. The discussion here is limited to some general remarks.

The therapist should keep the course of treatment as short as possible, compatible with the limits of tolerance and relief of symptoms. For instance, patients with brain metastases rarely survive longer than 6 months, and there seems little justification for spreading their treatment over several weeks. At the same time, although a large single treatment to the whole brain may give the same result, it may also produce cerebral oedema with unpleasant side effects. A suitable compromise is to fractionate therapy over 4 to 5 days.

Severe pain is often relieved with a short course of radiation therapy. If intractable pain persists, however, the therapist should consider other measures — the judicious use of analgesics and possibly neurosurgery, such as cordotomy.

Bleeding can often be controlled with small doses of radiation. Haemoptysis and haematuria from advanced cancer are specific indications for radiation. Fungating, malodorous growths may also respond to radiation, even in some so-called radioresistant tumours. The list of situations where palliative radiotherapy is of value is long, and it is recommended that the physician consult the therapist about individual problems as they arise.

EMERGENCIES

Early diagnosis and treatment is one of the cornerstones of cancer management. However, although all patients should be treated on an urgent basis, few true radiotherapeutic emergencies exist today. Even the most radio-sensitive tumours usually take several days to respond to radiation.

Acute haemorrhage is one emergency situation where radiotherapy may be of value. This is particularly important in a potentially curable disease, such as carcinoma of the cervix. Prompt institution of radium packing can often control the bleeding inside a few days. Catastrophic haemorrhage may require ligation of the hypogastric artery.

Spinal cord compression due to metastatic malignant disease should be treated immediately. The treatment of choice is laminectomy and surgical decompression. This should be followed as soon as possible by radiation therapy. This is particularly important in lesions with a good prognosis such as follicular thyroid cancer or Hodgkin's disease.

Respiratory obstruction is another rare situation where radiation therapy may be required urgently. When a patient with carcinoma of the larynx develops stridor, rapid initiation of treatment is essential. If symptoms worsen, facilities should be available for tracheostomy.

Superior vena caval obstruction usually responds rapidly to radiation. An obvious emergency exists when the patient presents with dyspnoea, cyanosis and papilloedema. Where radiation is not available a rapid response can often be obtained using steroids, diuretics and alkylating agents.

Patients with malignant disease involving the brain occasionally present in coma. Some of these patients have raised intracranial pressure and temporarily respond to steroids. Unfortunately many of these lesions represent metastatic disease but there are a few potentially curable situations. One of these is medulloblastoma where prompt treatment may be lifesaving.

AFTERCARE AND SIDE-EFFECTS

The radiotherapist must maintain a delicate balance between morbidity and mortality. With modern techniques radiation sickness is uncommon. However, radiation does produce inevitable side-effects in some anatomical sites. These include stomatitis, nausea, diarrhoea and dysuria. Side-effects can usually be anticipated and treated symptomatically. The patient should be warned beforehand and at the same time reassured that most of his symptoms will eventually subside. Late onset side-effects may give rise to more serious problems, such as fistula, necrosis and sometimes unexpected sequelae such as myxoedema.

Skilful application of radiotherapy produces excellent results with minimum morbidity. However, the indiscriminate use of radiation can cause extensive damage. The following list of side-effects is by no means complete:

Skin necrosis	Pulmonary fibrosis
Cataracts	Pericarditis
Xerostomia	Hepatitis
Transverse myelitis	Malabsorption syndrome
Thrombosis	Contracted bladder

Fractures	Sterility
Nephritis	Perichondritis
Aplastic anaemia	Growth deformity

FACTORS INFLUENCING RESULTS IN RADIOTHERAPY

1. STAGE. Generally this is the most important factor. The stage may be defined as the geographical extent of the disease. Several methods of staging have been described. None is entirely satisfactory although the TNM classification is widely used. T denotes the size of the tumour; N the presence of nodes; M represents distant metastases. The complete staging of a tumour can be approached in the following way:

a   Clinical staging from history and physical examination.
b   Investigations, eg, X-rays, laboratory tests, endoscopy, etc.
c   Surgical staging, eg, laparotomy in Hodgkin's disease.
d   Pathological staging.

2. RADIOSENSITIVITY AND GRADE. For a given stage, radiosensitive tumours have a better prognosis. This is partly to do with histological grade, but the relationship is complex.

3. LENGTH OF HISTORY. Stage for stage, a longer history has a worse prognosis in most forms of cancer. However, in some cases, the advantage of a short history may be offset by a more aggressive tumour.

4. SITE. Accessible tumours usually have a better prognosis, but this is often because of earlier diagnosis.

5. TUMOUR SIZE AND TUMOUR BED. Larger tumours require a bigger dose, but this is limited by the fact that large volumes of tissue tolerate radiation poorly. Vascularization of the tumour bed is also important. Thus friable exophytic tumours do better than indurated infiltrating lesions.

6. AGE. This has no effect by itself although the dose must often be reduced on account of poor circulation.

7. SEX. Prognosis is better in females for lesions of the head and neck. There is little difference in other sites.

8. ANAEMIA AND INFECTION. These reduce response to radiation.

9. DOSE. The optimum dose is usually the highest possible, compatible with an acceptable necrosis risk.

10. RADIOBIOLOGICAL FACTORS. Oxygenation is known to be important.

11. MISCELLANEOUS FACTORS. Radiotherapeutic response depends on the interplay of a large number of other factors, many of which are incompletely understood.

It has been shown however that treatment technique must be applied carefully each day, otherwise results will deteriorate.

FOLLOW-UP

Good patient management demands careful follow-up of all cases. There are many reasons for this:

1 Detection of residual disease.
2 Recognition of late recurrent disease.
3 Early side-effects. Patients need advice on how to cope with the immediate radiation reactions.
4 Late side-effects.
5 Detection of metastatic disease.
6 Detection of a second primary lesion. Many patients have a diathesis to certain forms of cancer.
7 Statistical assessment of results.

The spacing of follow-up appointments can be gauged according to the disease. Usually the patient is seen relatively frequently immediately following treatment, but longer intervals can be allowed later on. Follow-up appointments can be discontinued after a certain number of years, if the patient remains disease-free. This point occurs when the survival curve parallels that of the general population for the same age and sex.

References

Computers in Radiotherapy, Brit. J. Radiol., Special Report, Number 5, 1971.
Lowry, W. S. *The problem of alternative treatment days*, Clin. Radiol., 1972, **23**, 524.
Lowry, W. S. *The volume factor in radiotherapy. A new unit of dose: ret equivalent volume (rev.)*. Proceedings XIII International Radiological Congress, Madrid, 1973.
Meredith, W. J. *Radium dosage, The Manchester System*, Livingstone, London, 1967.
Paterson, R. *The treatment of malignant disease by radiotherapy*, Williams and Wilkins, Baltimore, 1963.
Quimby, E., and Castro, J. *Calculation of dosage in interstitial radium therapy*, Am. J. Roent., 1953, **70**, 739.
Shukovsky, L. J. *Dose, time, volume relationships in squamous cell carcinoma*, Am. J. Roent., 1970, **108**, 27.

6

Skin

Most malignant skin tumours are either basal cell carcinomas or squamous cell carcinomas. Rarer forms of skin cancer include malignant melanoma, lymphoma cutis, Kaposi's sarcoma and mycosis fungoides.

Aetiology

1. Actinic factors. Sunlight on exposed areas such as the face and hands. Pigmentation has a protective effect. Europeans living in tropical countries often develop skin cancer whereas negroes do not, apart from the very rare 'albino Bantu'.
2. Carcinogens. Hydrocarbons, pitch, tar, mineral oils (chimney sweep's cancer).
3. Ionizing radiation.
4. Arsenical keratosis.
5. Arising in chronically infected scars, eg, lupus vulgaris, gummas.

Pre-malignant Conditions

1. Hyperkeratosis.
2. Papillomas occasionally become malignant.
3. Xeroderma pigmentosum. Rare familial disease.
4. Leukoplakia at muco-cutaneous junctions.

Intra-epidermal Carcinoma *in situ*

1. Bowen's disease. This consists of multiple reddish-brown skin plaques. These are non-invasive but progressive.
2. Erythroplasia of Queyrat. This involves the mucous membranes of the mouth, glans and vulva.
3. Paget's disease of extra-mammary sites.

Invasive Cancer

I. BASAL CELL CARCINOMA (RODENT ULCER). Seventy-five per cent of cases. Commonly found on the face, above a line drawn between the angle of the mouth and lobe of the ear. Rarely seen on the ears. The lesions may be pigmented, 'wildfire', pearly or cystic. Histologically columns of cells grow solidly downwards from the basal layer. The disease rarely metastasizes unless there are squamous elements present. On palpation of the tumour there is often a central depression. A rare familial type called Gorlin's syndrome has been described.

2. SQUAMOUS CELL CARCINOMA. Twenty per cent of cases. This may occur anywhere on the body, but it is commonly found on the ear, lip and dorsum of the hand. The disease arises from stratified squamous epithelium or from metaplasia and is usually of multifocal origin. It is often possible to trace the various histological changes from the normal tissue edge, to overgrowth, to frank malignancy. Squamous carcinoma metastasizes along lymph channels.

3. MISCELLANEOUS SKIN CANCER. Rarely adenocarcinomas and basal cell lesions arise in sebaceous glands, sweat glands and hair follicles.

Treatment

Radiotherapy and surgery yield equally good results. Radiotherapy, however, is simple, involves no operation and gives a better cosmetic result. Superficial lesions can be adequately controlled by diathermy. Very superficial disease may sometimes be controlled with ointment impregnated with a cytotoxic agent, such as 5-fluorouracil.

SURGERY. The indications for surgery are as follows:

1 Lesions surrounded by areas of extensive premalignant change or leukoplakia.
2 Areas of reduced radiation tolerance, eg, perineum.
3 Scars from previous sepsis, surgery or syphilis.
4 Recurrence following radiotherapy.
5 Large lesions over 6 cm diameter. Sometimes radiotherapy may control a large bulky lesion where surgery is absolutely impossible.
6 Mobile lymph nodes.

Surgery may also be preferred in young patients, or in lesions involving bone, cartilage or tendon. Biopsy is usually essential to establish the diagnosis.

RADIOTHERAPY. (1) *Superficial X-ray therapy*. The treatment area should include an adequate margin of up to 1 cm of normal tissue around the tumour. The recommended dose is about 2100 rads in a single exposure or 3350 rads in 5 days. A better cosmetic result is claimed for more protracted therapy. Note that the proliferative part of the tumour will receive a higher dose if it projects in towards the X-ray source but this is not important. It has also been noted that some centres prescribe much higher doses. This is more apparent than real however since such treatment relates to soft or unfiltered low voltage radiation. Depth dose curves show that the dose below the epidermis is similar in both cases.

(2) *Radium mould*. This often gives an even better cosmetic result. The technique is preferred in regions of poor radiation tolerance overlying bone and cartilage (eg, ear and dorsum of hand). Radium combines the advantage of good quality radiation with the rapid fall-off in dose rate from a short source skin distance (SSD). The recommended skin dose is about 5500 rads in 7 days.

(3) *High energy radiation*. This is required for extensive skin lesions fixed to bone, eg, carcinoma of the ear extending on to the side of the head. The tumour should be 'waxed-up' with tissue equivalent material to allow irradiation of the skin surface. The dose depends on the size of the tumour, but it is usually necessary to extend fractionation over several weeks, eg 5000 rads in 3 weeks.

Fixed inoperable lymph nodes from skin carcinoma may sometimes respond to an extended course of megavoltage radiation. These results may be enhanced in the presence of high pressure oxygen.

Results

Five-year survival = 95 per cent.

One study suggests that there are two kinds of squamous carcinoma: the first, arising in hyperkeratotic lesions in Anglo-Saxon races, with a good prognosis; the second, arising *de nova* in other races, with a bad prognosis. There have also been reports of an increased incidence of skin cancer associated with other forms of malignancy such as lymphomas. In these situations the skin disease may be highly malignant and should be treated with special care and attention.

Complications

Following irradiation, patients develop an early skin reaction with erythema and epilation. This progresses to moist desquamation and can be treated with zinc and castor oil ointment if necessary. After 4 to 6 weeks a crust forms and the lesion heals.

Late radiation necrosis may develop after some years. This is more likely to occur in overlying cartilaginous areas. These lesions often respond to topical application of hydrocortisone ointment. Failing this, plastic surgery may be necessary.

Tumours of the canthi and eyelids carry special risks, and care should be taken to protect the lens. There is also an increased risk of ectropion, entropion and tear duct stenosis leaving a watering eye. For these reasons many therapists recommend surgery in this area.

KERATOACANTHOMA

This is not usually considered to be a form of skin cancer. However, its histological appearance is often indistinguishable from squamous cell carcinoma. Moreover on occasion it may behave in a highly malignant fashion. The tumour has a characteristic dome-shaped appearance. It normally grows explosively in a matter of a few weeks and then regresses spontaneously without treatment.

Some recent work suggests that perhaps keratoacanthoma and squamous cell carcinoma are the same disease, in a different host. In some patients the neoplasm provokes a brisk immunological response and is effectively rejected. In older patients, or those with immunoparesis, the disease may become frankly malignant. For this reason, if there is the slightest doubt about the nature of the tumour, it should be widely excised or treated with a radical course of superficial X-ray therapy. A suitable dose is 5500 rads in 3 weeks.

LYMPHOMA CUTIS

Any of the malignant lymphomas may involve skin, especially in the advanced stages. Primary involvement of the skin is extremely rare but does occur in a few cases. The term lymphoma cutis covers all these conditions. The lesions are radiosensitive and usually respond to moderate doses of superficial X-ray therapy, such as 3000 rads in 2 weeks. Treatment should be combined with systemic management of the disease. Prognosis is extremely variable, ranging from a few months to many years.

MYCOSIS FUNGOIDES

This disease is thought to be a primary malignant lymphoma involving the skin. Patients often have a long history of a chronic skin disease such as para-psoriasis or poilikoderma atrophicans vasculare. Multiple small scattered skin lesions eventually coalesce to form large characteristic thickened plaques.

The treatment of choice is superficial electron therapy. Again the disease usually responds to modest doses and may be controlled in this way for long periods of time. Superficial X-ray therapy is often satisfactory if electrons are not available. The disease is relatively slow growing, and patients usually survive for many years. However, over 50 per cent of all cases eventually develop a generalized form of lymphoma, often lymphosarcoma, and then require appropriate systemic management.

MALIGNANT MELANOMA

Aetiology

It is important to differentiate between simple melanosis and melanocytosis. Melanosis is increased pigmentation of the skin. Melanocytosis is an increase in the number of melanocytes. Benign and malignant varieties are recognized. The common intradermal mole or blue nevus is always benign. It is a hairy lesion and is not found on the palms, soles or scrotum. The compound or junctional nevus (between dermis and epidermis) is never hairy and is potentially malignant. Malignant melanoma may also develop spontaneously.

The cause of melanoma is unknown, but the relatively high rate of spontaneous regression suggests that immunological factors may sometimes be involved.

Pathology
There are no moles present at birth. Moles may, however, develop during infancy, but these are often junctional and the pathological diagnosis is sometimes difficult in this age group. Indeed junctional activity can be entirely normal before puberty.

The histological picture of melanoma varies from pleomorphism with bizarre giant cells to frank anaplasia. The cells may be amelanotic. The disease spreads by blood and lymph channels. Cutaneous spread with skin nodules is well recognized.

Classification
Three clinical varieties have been described:

1   Superficial spreading melanoma. The commonest type.
2   Nodular melanoma.
3   Lentigo malignum. Usually found on the faces of older patients.

Growth studies suggest that there is a very slow pre-pubertal form of melanoma with an 80 per cent 5-year survival. This form may recur after many years. There is also a fast variety that may kill inside a few weeks. This type is sometimes found in pregnancy, but the relationship may be coincidental.

Sites
Soles of feet (especially negroes).
Leg.
Nail bed.
Head and neck.
Retina (choroid and conjunctiva).
Meninges.
Mucous membranes (nose, mouth, gastro-intestinal tract, anus).

Treatment
(1) Radical surgery with wide excision and graft.
(2) Node dissection 2 weeks later. Some surgeons state that the prognosis is the same if one waits and dissects nodes if and when they appear.
(3) Juvenile melanomas developing before puberty have a frightening histology but often a good prognosis. Hence conservative surgery is sometimes advised for these cases.

(4) The disease is highly radioresistant. Radiotherapy is only indicated if the patient refuses surgery or there is a contra-indication to surgery. Radiation is mainly used palliatively to prevent fungation of malodorous inoperable lesions. Even for this purpose large doses of supervoltage radiation are required, up to 7000 rads in 7 weeks.

Experiments show that melanoma is radioresistant in tissue culture and has an increased 'shoulder'. If this can be exploited the disease may yet be made amenable to radiotherapy.

(5) Chemotherapy is reserved for advanced disease. Mitoclomine has been recommended in combination with other cytotoxic agents. Results are generally depressing although occasional long-term remissions have been reported.

(6) Immunotherapy. This is still experimental although some encouraging results have been obtained with BCG vaccination in a few cases.

Prognosis

Overall 5-year survival = 30 per cent.

The presence of several different types of disease confuses survival figures. However, the following factors affect prognosis:

1 Age: young patients do better and perhaps also very old patients.
2 Size: small early lesions have a good prognosis.
3 Sex: more benign in females.
4 Site: best in lower limb.
5 Type: lentigo malignum has a good prognosis. Nodular melanoma has a bad prognosis.

KAPOSI'S SARCOMA

Kaposi's sarcoma is a systemic disease which is usually confined to the skin in the early stages. Although the disease is rare in Britain and America, it is the commonest form of cancer in African negroes where it represents 10 per cent of all neoplasms. It has also been reported in other races.

The cause of Kaposi's sarcoma is unknown. The disease is mainly found in men. In Africa it is almost confined to the negro, even in areas where equivalent white, Indian and negro populations exist. Yet the condition is not familial.

Pathology

Some pathologists have suggested that it is a lymphoma; others suggest that it is a benign angiomatosis arising from multi-centric foci. But most pathologists believe it is a true sarcoma in which the secondary lesions are metastatic.

Histologically, Kaposi's sarcoma is a tumour of peri-vascular cells,

There are three phases in its development. The early cutaneous stage resembles an inflammatory reaction. This is followed by a granulomatous reaction associated with endothelial overgrowth forming vessel sinuses. The final stage is less vascular and resembles sarcoma.

Clinical Features

The disease usually presents as a skin condition starting on the legs. Tender raised hemispherical nodules about 1 cm diameter are found. These may become confluent. Later the nodules can either ulcerate or involute leaving a scar. Ten per cent of cases have visceral involvement, even in the absence of skin lesions. These are usually asymptomatic but may occasionally present as sudden haemorrhage. Ankle oedema is a sign of advanced disease. Soft tissue X-rays and angiograms may show deep-seated nodules. In the advanced stage there may be bony involvement resembling osteolytic sarcoma.

Treatment and Prognosis

Radiotherapy is the treatment of choice for early cases of Kaposi's sarcoma. Orthovoltage or megavoltage radiation may control local disease for long periods. The dose often has to be limited because of the large volume of tissue involved. In advanced cases, palliation has been obtained with extra-corporeal perfusion of nitrogen mustard.

The prognosis is not known with accuracy since there are no radiotherapy centres in many parts of Africa. Although follow-up studies are incomplete, one series did show an average overall survival of 8 years. There have also been a few cases of spontaneous regression.

Reference

M. D. Anderson Hospital. *Skin Cancer Symposium.* Yearbook Medical Publishers, Chicago, 1962.

Lowry, W. S., Hannemann, J. H., and Clark, D. *Skin Cancer and Immunosuppression*, 1972, Lancet, 1, 1290.

Rook, A., Wilkinson, D. S., and Ebling, F. J. G. *Textbook of Dermatology*, Blackwell, London, 1968.

7

Lip and Oral Cavity

CANCER OF THE LIP

This disease is commonly found in farmers exposed to the elements. Formerly there was an association with the smoking of clay pipes and with syphilis. A history of recurrent infection with herpes simplex may be obtained.

Most cases arise in the mucosa or vermilion border of the lower lip, halfway between the midline and the angle of the mouth. Typically a 'button'-like exophytic tumour with an indurated base is found. The rarer ulcerating infiltrating lesions tend to be more anaplastic.

Cancer of the lip drains to the sub-mental and sub-mandibular lymph glands. The tumour may cross the midline and metastasize to both sides of the neck. About 10 per cent of cases have nodes when first seen, and a further 10 per cent develop them later. Blood spread is unusual.

The much rarer tumour of the upper lip has a more extensive lymph drainage including the buccinator and pre-auricular nodes; it spreads more rapidly. There is a higher proportion of women with cancer of the upper lip.

The diagnosis must always be confirmed by biopsy. Serological examination should be made for syphilis.

Treatment

1. GENERAL MEASURES. Anaemia and dental sepsis should be corrected.

2. RADIOTHERAPY. This is the treatment of choice for most cases since the results are as good as surgery and the cosmetic appearance better. Superficial X-ray therapy may be used. Small fields of up to 3 × 2 cm are directed at the lip lesion. The nodes are not usually irradiated. A dose of about 2100 rads in a single exposure is adequate. Larger fractionated doses such as 3350 rads in 5 days or 5000 rads in 3 weeks give excellent cosmetic results. Somewhat smaller doses are recommended for elderly patients. A lead stent mould should be inserted in the buccal sulcus to protect the alveolus.

Good results may also be obtained using a two-plane or 'sandwich' radium mould. The recommended dose is 5500 rads in 8 days to the centre of the lesion and 7000 rads to the mucosa.

Careful follow-up at 2-monthly intervals for 2 years is vital. Very few patients develop metastases after this time.

3. SURGERY. Excision is usually reserved for patients with large lesions, for extensive leukoplakia, for recurrence following irradiation and for late radiation necrosis. Mobile lymph nodes should be removed by radical surgery. If the nodes are fixed to the mandible, then the mandible itself should be removed. Prophylactic lymph node dissection is not recommended since results appear to be as good if a watching policy is adopted.

Results
The 5-year survival is 95 per cent. Even with palpable lymph nodes the 5-year survival is 50 per cent. With bilateral nodes the survival has fallen to 25 per cent. The overall 5-year survival for upper lip cancer is 50 per cent.

Complications
A late radiation reaction may develop many years after radiotherapy. This can often be controlled by topical application of steroids in emollient dental paste. Radiation necrosis occurs in up to 10 per cent of cases. This does not alter prognosis but it does require plastic repair.

CANCER OF THE MOUTH
General Remarks
The treatment at specific anatomical sites is considered below but some general comments apply to this area.

The incidence of cancer of the mouth is steadily declining, and the relative preponderance of males to females is disappearing. This is mainly due to better dental hygiene and earlier treatment of syphilis. Cancer in the tonsillar area is increasing relative to cancer in other sites in the head and neck and is related to alcoholism. Smoking is also an important aetiological factor. In Asian countries, oral cancer is associated with betel nut chewing and the custom of 'reverse' smoking.

Histologically, squamous cell carcinomas are seen in varying degrees of differentiation. Around the tumour there is often a surrounding area of pre-malignant leukoplakia. The prognosis depends on the anatomical site. The more posterior the lesion, the worse the prognosis.

The management of oral cancer illustrates the importance of a combined therapeutic attack on this disease. Generally the treatment of choice is radiotherapy to the primary tumour, followed by a radical dissection of palpable lymph nodes in the neck. Pre-operative radiation is also used extensively.

External Radiotherapy

Supervoltage therapy alone may control the disease in some cases. The treatment fields should include the primary lesion and the lymph node drainage areas in the neck.

The dose to the primary lesion varies depending on the extent of the disease, from 5500 rads in 5 weeks to 7000 rads in 7 weeks. If a radical neck dissection is planned later, the recommended dose to the neck should not exceed 4500 rads. Additional therapy to the primary lesion can then be given through reduced fields.

Supervoltage techniques often involve treating the patient through two parallel opposed portals, with the dose weighted 2 to 1 towards the diseased side. Care must be taken to avoid excessive irradiation of the cervical cord. Accurate dosimetry may sometimes call for the use of rotation therapy, wedge fields, or electrons.

Dental sepsis should be treated beforehand since extractions in the irradiated areas lead to complications. Complete dental clearance is sometimes necessary, especially in lesions of the alveolus.

Interstitial Therapy

Small localized lesions are often best treated with radium needle or radon seed implant. A portable image intensifier at the operation enables radiographic control, and errors of needle distribution can be corrected immediately. The involved zone should be treated together with the surrounding margin of normal tissue. The recommended dose is about 6000 rads in 7 days. This dose may be reduced slightly for areas over 20 sq. cm and increased for areas under 9 sq. cm. For further details of radium technique and dosimetry the reader is referred to several reference works on the subject.

A combination of supervoltage therapy and interstitial therapy is sometimes recommended in selected cases. The technique involves giving an external dose of 4500 rads in four and a half weeks to the primary and node-bearing areas followed by an interstitial implant to the primary lesion to a dose of 2500 rads in 3 days. This enables one to deliver a highly effective dose to the primary tumour and, at the same time, adequately irradiate the marginal areas.

Surgery

Surgery is often indicated in the treatment of well-differentiated tumours which are less radiosensitive than undifferentiated tumours. Bone invasion is also an indication for primary surgery although pre-operative radiation often improves survival.

Bilateral block dissection of the neck is the treatment of choice for mobile neck nodes. It consists in removal of all soft tissue between the platysma and the pre-scalene fascia in both triangles of the neck. This includes all lymphatic tissue and the jugular vein, but spares the carotid artery and the vagus nerve. The contents are removed *en bloc* from the mandible above to the clavicle below. Complete resection of the tumour with a radical dissection of the neck and removal of the intervening structures in continuity — the so-called 'commando' operation — is a mutilating procedure but has a limited place in the treatment of oral cancer.

Fixed Neck Nodes

Fixed inoperable metastatic lymph nodes in the neck create a difficult therapeutic problem. A course of external radiation therapy to a dose of 4500 rads in four and a half weeks is sometimes recommended. Six weeks later such nodes may become mobile and operable. In recent years a more aggressive radiotherapeutic approach to the problem of fixed neck nodes has been taken. Several techniques have been tried. These include multiple split course therapy, irradiation in hyperbaric oxygen and a combination of supervoltage therapy followed by a small localized interstitial implant.

Radiation Reactions

Radiation reactions in the mouth develop in all cases. Patients are advised to stop smoking and to avoid hot and cold fluids and alcoholic spirits. Viscous Xylocaine is sometimes necessary to control severe mucositis. Occasionally superimposed infections may develop, including monilia. Fortunately, however, the good blood supply of the mouth usually ensures rapid healing.

The salivary glands are often damaged. The serous acini are more affected than the mucous glands, and saliva becomes thick and sticky. Patients also complain of loss of taste sensation. Some return of function occurs in most cases.

Xerostomia damages the teeth leading to brown discoloration, caries and generalized superficial defects. There may also be damage to the periodontal membrane leading to loosening of the teeth.

Painful ulcers may develop on the soft parts of the mouth. If these do not heal spontaneously, electro-coagulation may be required. Bone pain can occur with no overlying skin defect. In this case, it is advisable to wait until the sequestrum separates spontaneously. Severe osteonecrosis may necessitate hemi-mandibulectomy. Salivary fistulae may require plastic surgery.

CARCINOMA OF ANTERIOR TWO-THIRDS OF TONGUE

Eighty-five per cent of lesions occur at the edge of the tongue, 10 per cent at the tip and 4 per cent on the dorsum. The tumour spreads directly through the tongue and floor of the mouth. One-third of cases have lymph node metastases when first seen and a further third develop nodes later, usually in the deep cervical chain.

Clinical Features

Lump or ulcer.

Pain in ear or tongue.

Speech difficulty — tongue stuck to floor of mouth.

Dysphagia.

Neck swelling.

Treatment

RADIOTHERAPY. This is the treatment of choice for most cases. Small flat lesions may be treated with a radioactive gold seed implant; lesions on the lateral border with a vertical plane radium implant, and lesions on the dorsum with a horizontal plane implant. Large bulky infiltrating lesions may be treated with a radium needle volume implant. The tongue is usually stitched to the floor of the mouth during treatment. More extensive lesions may require external megavoltage radiation or combination therapy as outlined above.

SURGERY. Surgery is indicated in the following cases:

1 Carcinoma complicating syphilis. Here the disease is often extensive and the vascular supply destroyed.

2 Small lesions on tip of tongue.

3 Recurrence after radiotherapy.

4 Leukoplakia. The growth should be excised along with the affected mucosa on the dorsum of the tongue.

5 Lymph node metastases.

Prognosis

Five-year survival = 25 per cent.

FLOOR OF MOUTH

This disease behaves in much the same way as carcinoma of the tongue. Surgery is indicated if the gum is invaded or the lingual nerve involved. In these cases the prognosis following irradiation is poor, and a limited operative approach sometimes enables the surgeon to preserve the anterior mandibular arch for subsequent repair.

For smaller lesions a two plane radium needle implant or a double radium mould may be used. Supervoltage radiation may be used for larger tumours.

The 5-year survival is 40 per cent.

LOWER ALVEOLUS

This tumour spreads locally to the cheek, medially to the floor of the mouth, downwards to the mandible and backwards to the anterior tonsillar pillar and pterygo-maxillary region. The mental foramen is often invaded, especially if the patient is edentulous. Sixty-five per cent of cases develop nodes at some stage. Lymph drainage is to the sub-mental, sub-mandibular and upper deep cervical nodes.

Clinically this tumour presents with bleeding, ill-fitting dentures, pain, otalgia and trismus.

Early cases with superficial erosion of the mandible may be treated by a radium mould. Moderately advanced cases with invasion of the mandible should be widely resected along with neck nodes.

Advanced cases should be treated by external megavoltage radiation.

The 5-year survival is 30 per cent.

UPPER ALVEOLUS

This very rare tumour spreads up to the maxillary antrum, outwards to the cheek, medially to the palate and posteriorly to the anterior tonsillar pillar and pterygo-maxillary region. Most lesions are squamous carcinomas but occasionally intra-oral melanoma is seen. Lymph channels drain to the anterior jugular region and rarely to the sub-mandibular and upper deep cervical nodes. Nodes are palpable in 40 per cent of cases. Carcinoma of the antrum is an important differential diagnosis.

Again the disease may present with pain, ill-fitting dentures, bleeding and trismus.

Small superficial lesions can be treated by an intra-oral radium mould. Larger lesions may require external megavoltage therapy. More extensive lesions invading bone may necessitate resection of the maxilla.

The 5-year survival is 40 per cent.

CARCINOMA OF THE PALATE

Some differences between hard and soft palate tumours are outlined in Table IX. The clinical features are similar to those outlined above although advanced cases may develop dysphagia.

TABLE IX

Comparison of carcinoma of hard and soft palate

	Soft palate	Hard palate
Incidence	Three times more common	—
Sex ratio	Males = females	Males greater than females
Spread	Retropharyngeal and upper deep cervical nodes	Ditto plus submandibular nodes
Metastases	60 per cent nodes	30 per cent nodes
Treatment	Often radiotherapy	Often surgery
Prognosis	20 per cent cure	50 per cent cure

Salivary and mucous gland neoplasms are slightly more common than squamous carcinoma in the palate. It is important to exclude primary tumours of the antrum, nasopharynx or upper jaw presenting at the palate.

Superficial lesions with minimal infiltration may be treated by a gold seed implant for the soft palate, or a radium mould for the hard palate. Medium-sized lesions of the hard palate and those associated with leuko-plakia require surgery. Advanced lesions can sometimes be controlled with external megavoltage radiation.

TONSILLAR AREA

This region includes the palatine arch, the posterior faucial pillars, the tonsillar fossa, the glossopalatine sulcus, the pharyngeal wall and the base of the tongue. The palatine arch consists of a small amount of mucous membrane stretched over the ascending mandibular ramus (retro-molar triangle), the anterior faucial pillar and the central soft palate and uvula. Tumours originating in these various anatomical sites follow different clinical patterns.

Most of the lesions are squamous cell carcinomas. The second com-monest lesion is a lymphoma which is usually a reticulum cell sarcoma. Ectopic salivary gland tumours have also been noted. Usually squamous cell carcinomas are well differentiated when they originate on the palatine arch but are anaplastic when they originate in the tonsillar fossa or the glosso-palatine sulcus.

Patients usually present with a sore throat, dysphagia or a lump in the neck.

Patients with lesions of the palatine arch have a 50 per cent incidence of clinically positive neck nodes when first seen, whereas in patients with primary lesions in the tonsillar fossa or glossopalatine sulcus the incidence is 70 per cent. Moreover in the patients with lesions in the tonsillar fossa, the nodes are often multiple, fixed or bilateral. Patients with lesions of the palatine arch develop symptoms earlier because of dysphagia but those with lesions in the tonsillar fossa or glossopalatine sulcus usually present with neck nodes.

Treatment

Early tumours of the palatine arch should be treated with radiotherapy. The portals should cover the primary lesion, the sub-digastric area at the angle of the jaw which is the commonest site for a single node.

When the disease involves bone or infiltrates deeply into the pterygoid space, surgery is preferred. If this invasive type of lesion is irradiated, the incidence of local failure is high. Attempts to salvage such patients by radical resection after radiotherapy are fraught with severe complications, including rupture of the carotid artery.

Most cases of cancer of the tonsillar fossa should be treated by radiotherapy. The primary lesion usually responds well to treatment. The treatment fields should include the primary site and the neck. Occasionally the dose to the tonsillar area can be boosted with a gold seed implant. The whole neck is irradiated pre-operatively when there are multiple nodes. The recommended dose levels were given earlier in the general discussion on oral cancer.

If a radical neck dissection is planned later, then a bifurcate incision is recommended. This prevents the complications seen with the usual trifurcate incision, which invariably has its apex over the carotid artery. Irradiation failures of lesions originating on the palatine arch can often be salvaged. But those of the tonsillar fossa or glossopalatine sulcus are rarely excised because of the more inaccessible location.

Results
Five-year survivals of 20 per cent were previously recorded but, with the more aggressive treatment outlined above, some centres claim that this figure can be increased to over 50 per cent.

BUCCAL MUCOSA
This disease is usually detected relatively early and consequently has a better prognosis. Small lesions may be amenable to an interstitial implant. More advanced disease requires external irradiation. Surgery is indicated where the mandible or nodes are involved. The dose patterns are similar to those outlined above.

Reference

Paterson, R. *The treatment of malignant disease by radiotherapy*, Williams and Wilkins, Baltimore, 1963.

8

Ear, Nose and Throat

MIDDLE EAR

Carcinoma of the middle ear is a relatively rare disease. Chronic otitis media is a recognized predisposing factor. Cancer may also develop in an old scar or sinus.

Cholesteatoma is a pre-malignant condition. This is not a true tumour but an overgrowth of squamous epithelium. (*Note.* Squamous epithelium is not normally present in the middle ear. It arises because of chronic infection and squamous metaplasia.)

Pathology

Squamous carcinoma, 90 per cent.
Glomus jugulare, 5 per cent. (See Chemodectoma.)
Miscellaneous, eg, melanoma, basal cell carcinoma, etc, 5 per cent.

The tumour is confined by bone and local spread is slow. Eventually the disease extends into the petrous portion of the temporal bone and middle cranial fossa. It also extends outwards to the surface of the skull. In 10 per cent of cases, lymphatic spread occurs to the upper deep cervical, retropharyngeal and pre-auricular nodes.

Clinical Features

The main symptoms and signs are pain, discharge, deafness and VIIth nerve paralysis. Late features include lymph node swelling, meningeal irritation and abscess. The tumour may perforate the tympanic membrane and present as a swelling at the external meatus.

Investigations

1 X-ray for petrous bone destruction (sub-mento occipital view).
2 Biopsy. Repeat frequently if necessary, especially where there is chronic granulation tissue in a suppurative ear.

Treatment

This is based on the extent of the disease and the patient's general condition. There is usually an element of infection requiring antibiotic therapy.

C

RADIOTHERAPY. Megavoltage therapy is recommended. Wedge fields 5 × 5 cm are often convenient. If the skin is involved, the surface is 'waxed-up' with tissue equivalent material to build up the surface dose. Alternatively a direct field short SSD Caesium 137 beam may be used to a depth of 5 cm. Electron beam therapy has also been recommended; a suitable dose is 5500 rads in 3 weeks.

SURGERY. This allows biopsy and drainage. Surgical exposure also reveals the full extent of the disease. Combinations of surgery and radiotherapy have been recommended in some centres. However, radical removal of the temporal bone is a formidable procedure and is rarely justified.

The nursing care is an important part of surgical management. The deep bony cavity should be kept clean and crusting periodically removed until the area is fully epithelialized.

Results
Radiotherapy alone gives 5-year survival rates of 30 per cent. Recurrence is rare after 2 years. Surgery alone has a higher morbidity and lower survival rate. Combination therapy has yet to be evaluated.

Palliation is disappointing because pain is difficult to relieve until the lesion has fully healed. Furthermore, even following cure, pain may take a long time to clear.

Complications
1   Infection.
2   Bone necrosis. Sequestra should be allowed to separate and should not be excised.
3   Brain abscess.
4   Poor beam direction can result in brain damage and transverse myelitis.

CHEMODECTOMA
This rare tumour arises from non-chromaffin paraganglia chemoreceptor cells. It is associated with parasympathetic nerves and starts in the adventitia of blood vessels around efferent nerves, mainly along branches of the glosso-pharyngeal and vagus nerves or their ganglions.

Sites
Most tumours are found in the dome of the jugular bulb (glomus jugulare) under the floor of the middle ear, the glomus body of the temporal bone or in the carotid body. A large number of other sites have been described including the auricular branch of the vagus, the aortic body, the femoral artery and the ciliary ganglion of the orbit. These tumours should not be confused

with either the exquisitely tender glomus tumours of the nail bed, or chromaffin tumours of the adrenal.

Chemodectomas are locally invasive and rarely metastasize. They are usually found in middle-aged females who may present with tinnitus, deafness or vertigo. Calcification may be noted on X-ray, but the diagnosis usually necessitates angiogram, best seen in the venous phase.

Treatment

Radiotherapy is recommended for tumours of the glomus jugulare. Treatment may prevent invasion of the petrous parts of the temporal bone. The recommended dose is 5000 rads in 3 weeks using wedge filters. Fields should extend to a depth of 2 cm from the midline of the skull. Biopsy of this vascular tumour is dangerous and may result in torrential haemorrhage.

Surgery is usually reserved for carotid body tumours where bleeding may be more easily controlled. Radiotherapy may be tried if surgery is not feasible or if excision is inadequate.

The overall results of treatment are excellent with 5-year survivals of over 80 per cent.

AIR SINUSES: MAXILLARY ANTRUM

Cancer may develop in the upper or lower half of the antrum. Tumours of the infrastructure are more common and often present at the palate. Suprastructure lesions usually develop at the upper inner angle of the antrum. These tumours spread rapidly to the ethmoids and nasal cavity.

Aetiology

Chronic maxillary sinusitis is a predisposing factor. The disease has been found in woodworkers in the furniture industry. It also is common in Africa. The reasons for this are unknown.

Pathology

Ninety per cent of lesions are squamous carcinomas in varying degrees of differentiation. Rarer tumours include lymphosarcoma, adamantinoma, cylindroma, unpigmented melanoma and plasmacytoma.

The clinical features depend on the spread of the disease which may be:

1 Anterior into the face.
2 Inferior into the palate. (Do not misdiagnose as primary carcinoma of the palate.)
3 Medially to the nasal cavity.
4 Backwards to the zygoma and pterygoid muscles giving trismus.
5 Upwards into the orbit giving proptosis and cranial nerve involvement.

6   Lymphatic spread to the upper deep cervical, retropharyngeal and sub-mandibular nodes in 30 per cent of cases.

Investigations
1   X-rays, including laminograms (base view).
2   Cytology. Antral washings are examined for malignant cells.
3   Biopsy — see below.
4   Test vision of both eyes. Sacrifice of the ipsilateral eye may be necessary.

Treatment
A decision on radical or palliative therapy is made depending on the extent of the disease and the general condition of the patient. With surgery or radiotherapy alone results are disappointing. The following combination has been recommended in some centres.

(1) Wide open permanent sinusostomy through the hard palate or canine fossa. This allows biopsy, drainage and antibiotic therapy. Dental sepsis should be treated at the same time.

(2) Supervoltage therapy up to a dose of 5500 rads in 5 weeks. Wedge field arrangements about 7 × 7 cm are used avoiding the opposite eye.

The field should normally extend:

a   Above to the supra-orbital ridge.
b   Below to the upper alveolus.
c   Medially to 1 cm on opposite side of nasal septum.
d   Backwards to posterior limb of infra-temporal fossa.

If the disease is early and confined to the infrastructure, it may be possible to save the eye. In this case the patient is asked to look upwards during treatment, and the upper edge of the anterior field is kept just below the cornea and pupil.

A 'biteblock' in the mouth avoids an air space and keeps the tongue clear of the treatment fields. The skin is 'waxed-up' if involved.

(3) Transpalatal surgery 6 weeks later. If the suprastructure is involved, radical maxillectomy is advised, opening the antrum and ethmoids into a single cavity. This may be followed by orbital exenteration if indicated.

(4) If the disease is still active on microscopy, then an intracavitary applicator or gold implant may be necessary.

(5) Involved nodes may be dissected or treated with radiation if inaccessible.

(6) The palate defect is filled with an obturator.

Results
The 5-year survival is 25 per cent. Some series claim 40 per cent with the above combined approach.

ETHMOID, SPHENOID AND FRONTAL SINUSES

These neoplasms have generally similar features to cancer of the antrum except that they are rarer and the prognosis poorer. If the eye is in the treatment field it can be 'waxed-up'. A peephole can then be left, and the patient told to look into the X-ray set. In this way a certain amount of protection is given to the anterior chamber.

Palliation is disappointing, and one should attempt to cure each case with a radical dose if possible. If the patient's condition is hopeless, the eyes can be protected and a single exposure of 1250 rads may provide useful palliation although protracted treatment may be better tolerated.

NASAL FOSSA

Primary tumours are rare. Secondary spread is usually from the antrum, ethmoid sinus or nasopharynx.

Histology
1 Squamous carcinoma, 90 per cent.
2 Lymphosarcoma.
3 Salivary gland tumour.
4 Extramedullary plasmacytoma (commonest site).
5 Rhabdomyosarcoma.
6 Esthesio-neuroepithelioma (olfactory neuroblastoma).
7 Malignant granuloma.

Clinical Features
The commonest symptoms are nasal obstruction and a bloody mucous nasal discharge. Patients may also have symptoms due to local extension and lymph spread.

Investigations
1 Anterior and posterior rhinoscopy using 0·5 per cent cocaine to obtain shrinkage of mucosa.
2 X-rays and tomograms may show a cloudy antrum and antral wall involvement.
3 Biopsy.

Treatment
Small tumours may be treated with a radon seed implant.

Tumours of the vestibule, lower conchae, floor and lower septum may be treated on megavoltage by a pair of wedge fields 4 × 4 cm. If the fields are very small, a dose of up to 6000 rads in 3 weeks can be given.

In the upper nasal cavity the prognosis is poorer. In these cases combination of radical radiotherapy and surgery is advised where possible.

Results

The prognosis is variable and depends on the exact site and extent of the disease.

Malignant Granuloma of the Nose

This lesion is sometimes called lethal midline granuloma. This is not a true cancer and may be associated with Wegener's disease and polyarteritis nodosa. The destructive granulomatous process is probably due to localized 'hyper-immunity'. The lesion progresses to ulceration, bone necrosis and gangrene. Low dosage radiation to about 1000 rads often provides local control. Steroids may also be given.

NASOPHARYNX

Histology

1   Sixty per cent are epithelial tumours variously described as squamous carcinoma and 'transitional' cell carcinoma.
2   Thirty-five per cent are lymphoma or lympho-epithelioma. These lesions are derived from adenoid lymph tissue. They are usually found in young people.
3   Miscellaneous.

Spread

The roof of the nasopharynx is the floor of the sphenoid sinus. There are no lateral or superior barriers to spread, and 25 per cent of tumours extend through the base of the skull. They also spread laterally to the pterygoid fossa and anteriorly to the nasal mucosa.

Ninety per cent of cases have lymph spread to the retropharyngeal or deep cervical nodes.

Clinical Features

An adult with no previous ear trouble and a persistent unilateral serous otitis media should be observed very carefully for carcinoma of the naso-pharynx. Other clinical features include neck swelling, deafness due to fluid in the ear and cranial nerve palsy.

Investigations

Tumours of the nasopharynx are notoriously difficult to diagnose.

1   Mirror examination. This may be negative even with cranial nerve involvement.
2   Biopsy. Repeated random punch biopsy is often necessary.
3   X-rays.
    a   Sub-mento vertical. This may show invasion of the base of skull.

    b   Lateral soft tissue film.

    c   Frontal and sagittal tomograms may be the only way of visualizing the neoplasm. Ethmoid extension or destruction of the basi-sphenoid may be seen.

4   Nasopharyngoscope.

Treatment

Megavoltage therapy. Two laterally opposed fields are used. The recommended dose is up to 7000 rads in 7 weeks. Smaller doses suffice in lymphomas. The fields should be as small as possible but must include the following regions: the nasopharynx; the base of the skull including the sphenoid sinus; the lymphatics in the posterior wall of the pharynx; the upper neck lymph nodes down to the thyroid notch.

The posterior edge of the field should be tilted backwards 5 degrees to include the posterior wall of the nasopharynx. It has been stated that this angle is critical and that a 10 degree tilt will catch the spinal cord. Verification films should be taken. The ear flap can often be protected.

Results

Thirty per cent overall 5-year survival (even with nodes).

Fifty per cent for lymphoma.

If the cranial nerves or the base of skull are involved the prognosis is poor.

Complications

1   Dental sepsis. Carious teeth should be extracted beforehand.
2   Otitis media.
3   Radiation myelitis. The total dose to the cervical cord must not exceed 5000 rads.
4   Xerostomia.
5   Chronic external otitis.

OROPHARYNX

The pharyngeal walls are considered here. For the tonsillar region, see the sections on the mouth (Chapter 7).

Pathology

The lesion is usually squamous carcinoma.

The disease spreads locally to the base of the skull, the eustachean tube, the palate and the mandible.

Lymph spread to retropharyngeal nodes occurs in 45 per cent of cases. It may also spread to the internal jugular chain.

Investigations
1 Biopsy.
2 X-ray lateral soft tissue view of neck to assess the upper and lower extension of the disease.

Clinical Features
Cancer of the pharynx usually presents with pain and dysphagia. This leads to loss of weight and eventual emaciation. Often patients have neck nodes when they are first seen.

Treatment
Surgical resection is the treatment of choice where possible.

Radiotherapy is reserved for very small exophytic growths. A dose of up to 5000 rads in 5 weeks can be given. Radiotherapy is not recommended for advanced lesions. In these cases the scanty pre-vertebral fascia often fails to heal.

Results
Very poor.

LARYNX

Sites
1 Glottis (superior surface and edge of true cords). Seventy per cent of cases.
2 Supra-glottic (false cords and ventricle). Twenty per cent.
3 Sub-glottic (inferior surface cords). Ten per cent.

Aetiology
Chronic laryngitis, smoking, singing and alcohol are predisposing factors. The disease has also been seen in industrial workers exposed to wood and metal dust. Cancer of the larynx is rare in women.

Pathology
Papilliferous, proliferative and nodular types of tumours are common. The membranous ulcerative type is rare and has a poor prognosis.

Ninety-nine per cent of cases are squamous carcinoma. These are usually keratinized and well differentiated.

Local growth is slow, and most early cord lesions have no metastases. Direct spread occurs across the anterior commissure to the opposite cord. Fixation of the cord often means there is muscle infiltration. Later there is extension to the supra- and sub-glottic regions. Lymphatic spread occurs late. The free edge of the true cord has no lymphatics, but nearly sub-mucous lymphatics drain to the deep cervical nodes. Blood-borne metastases are unusual.

Clinical Features
Hoarseness, loss of voice, dry cough and neck swelling are the main present-ing symptoms. Haemoptysis, dysphagia, stridor, dyspnoea and pain are late features.

Investigations
1   Laryngoscopy, indirect and direct with biopsy.
2   Serology for syphilis.
3   X-ray chest, soft tissue view of neck, tomogram and laryngogram.

Stage
   o   Pre-malignant leukoplakia and hyperkeratosis.
   I   Limited to mucous membrane (mobile larynx).
   II   Early and late cord fixation.
   III   Growth beyond larynx and/or mobile neck nodes.
   IV   Fixed nodes and/or skin involvement and/or distant metastases.

Treatment
In deciding between surgery or radiotherapy one should consider the patient's age, occupation and personality. Anaemia and sepsis should be corrected.

RADIOTHERAPY. This is recommended for early and late cases. Megavoltage radiation using Cobalt 60 teletherapy preferably with a short SSD is advised. Lateral parallel opposed or wedged fields about 7×5 cm are used. Occasion-ally a small unilateral lesion can be treated with a single field about 4×4 cm on the involved side. Bulky lesions require large field sizes, but these can be reduced during the last quarter of treatment. The posterior edges of fields should be kept in front of the transverse processes of the vertebral bodies. The usual prescribed dose is about 6000 rads in 5 to 6 weeks. Some therapists recommend 5500 rads in 3 to 4 weeks to the smaller fields.

The question of when to treat pre-malignant disease is unsettled. If one elects to use radiation, a full dose should be given since retreatment is not possible later.

Patients should be advised not to talk or smoke during treatment. Antibiotics and analgesics are prescribed as required.

SURGERY. Operation is reserved for Stage II and III cases including complete cord fixation, cartilage invasion and for perichondritis and irradia-tion failures. It is also indicated for patients who are unable to lie still, eg, Parkinson's disease, and where follow-up facilities are inadequate, eg, patients living in remote country areas. The following surgical procedures have been used:
1   Total or hemi-laryngectomy.
2   Fenestration (Finzi-Harmer). Radium needles are then inserted through a window cut in thyroid cartilage. Not often used today.
3   Laryngo-fissure excision with partial laryngectomy.

PRE-OPERATIVE RADIATION. This is given in many centres for inter-mediate cases. The recommended dose is 4500 rads in 4 to 5 weeks. A 6-week gap is allowed for recovery prior to surgery.

NODES. Mobile nodes call for neck dissection. Radiotherapy also gives good results in some of these cases, although this fact is not widely appreciated. Large fields can be used to include the primary lesion and the drainage pathways.

Fixed nodes may be treated with megavoltage therapy. High pressure oxygen irradiation may improve results in these advanced cases.

Results
The 5-year survival is 80 per cent for glottis. Twenty-five per cent survival is quoted for supra-and sub-glottic regions. Most patients regain their voice following radiotherapy, whereas total laryngectomy leaves the patient with oesophageal speech.

Complications
An early skin reaction and pharyngitis are usual. The airway may be threatened by laryngeal oedema necessitating tracheostomy.

Late side-effects include vocal cord damage with telangiectasia and cornification. Chronic cough with phlegm may also occur. Pain and dysphagia from perichondritis have been noted in some cases. Transverse myelitis is a rare complication and should not be seen with the better geometrical alignment of patients today.

EXTRINSIC LARYNX
Epilaryngeal
This area includes the supra-hyoid epiglottis, arytenoid cartilages and ary-epiglottic folds. Patients often complain of pain on swallowing. Nodes appear early. Equally good results are obtained with pharyngo-laryngectomy or megavoltage therapy. Lesions at the tip of the epiglottis have a good prognosis. Lower down the prognosis worsens.

Hypopharynx or Post-cricoid Carcinoma
These lesions are often found in women associated with the Plummer-Vinson syndrome. External radiation to a radical dose level is recommended. The 5-year survival is 20 per cent. Surgical results are also disappointing.

Pyriform Fossa
The lesion is often squamous carcinoma and is associated with alcoholism. It usually occurs in men. Neck nodes may be quite large before the primary lesion is visible. An aggressive approach with combined surgery and mega-

voltage radiotherapy is indicated. The prognosis has improved recently and 5-year survival rates between 30 and 50 per cent have been quoted.

UNKNOWN PRIMARY

Occasionally patients present with carcinoma in a neck node and no primary site can be found. Some of these tumours originate from occult primary lesions in the nasopharynx, laryngopharynx or lung. In alcoholic patients the primary site may be in the upper food passages.

An aggressive radiotherapeutic approach is warranted in these cases with supervoltage therapy to a dose of at least 5000 rads in 5 weeks.

The 5-year survival is 30 per cent for surgery and 50 per cent for radiotherapy. The increased survival following irradiation may be because the treatment portals sometimes encompass the primary disease.

References

Fechner, R. F., and Lamppin, J. *Midline Granuloma*, Arch. Otolaryngol., 1972, **95**, 467.

Harrison, D. F. B. *Carcinoma of the larynx*, Brit. Med. J., 1969, 615.

Lott, S., and Hazrat, T. *Carcinoma of the larynx*, John Hopkins Med. J., 1972, **4**, 244.

Morrison, R. *Radiation therapy in diseases of the larynx*, Review article, Brit. J. Radiol., 1971, **44**, 289.

9

Orbit and Salivary Glands

THE EYE

Skin cancer on or near the eyelids is discussed in Chapter 6.

It is worth recalling the anatomical measurements of the eye. The orbit can be considered as a cone or pyramid 4 cm high with a base 4 cm diameter. The globe is 2·5 cm diameter. The lens is 5 mm deep to the cornea which is 1 mm thick.

Tumours may arise from any of the contents of the orbit including the eye, optic nerve and lacrimal gland. They may also arise from structures forming the orbit, eg, muscle, giving rhabdomyosarcoma. Tumours of nearby structures, eg, nose, may invade the orbit. A tumour may also be part of a generalized disease process such as metastatic breast carcinoma. Occasionally lymphosarcoma of the orbit is seen.

The common primary neoplasms of the eye are malignant melanoma and retinoblastoma.

The following stages are recognized:

  I   Globe.
 II   Orbit.
III   Metastases.

MALIGNANT MELANOMA*

Melanin cells are found in the uveal tract, ie, choroid, ciliary body and iris, and malignant melanoma may arise in any of these sites. The disease is often anaplastic, and there is usually early invasion of the surrounding tissue. The course of the disease is extremely variable and following apparently successful removal, metastases can be discovered up to 10 years later. This has given rise to the clinical axiom, 'beware of the man with the glass eye and the enlarged liver'.

Clinically the patient usually presents with a scotoma associated with a detached retina. However, it is possible to have a moderate-sized lesion

* See also Chapter 6.

without being aware of it, and periodic eye examinations in adults are often recommended for this reason.

Treatment

1 Enucleation with orbital exenteration. It is necessary to remove the orbital periosteum to obtain a good result.
2 Post-operative radiation is given if there is residual tumour present or if there is recurrence following surgery. A dose of 5500 rads in 3 weeks is recommended using small 5 × 5 cm wedged fields.
3 Glass prosthesis.

Difficulty arises if the patient has only one eye. In these cases vision may sometimes be preserved if less than one quarter of the retina has been destroyed, or if the lesion measures less than 10 mm diameter. The eye is exposed at operation, and a small disc of Cobalt 60 sewn on to the affected area. The dosimetry is arranged so that the base of the lesion receives 40 000 rads and the summit 14 000 rads. At the end of treatment the disc is removed.

Results

Five-year survival = 50 per cent.

CANCEROUS MELANOSIS OF THE CONJUNCTIVA

Unlike melanoma, this disease is radiosensitive. Surgical excision is recommended if the lids are involved. If the lesion is near the limbus, exuberant masses should be excised to obtain a flat surface. Thereafter small lesions can be treated with a Strontium 90 beta plaque to a dose of 2000 rads per week for 4 weeks. If the entire conjunctival sac is involved, a radon seed ring can be sewn around the globe. The bulbar and lid conjunctiva are then treated to a dose of 4000 rads in 4 days. More extensive lesions require X-ray therapy. The overall prognosis for these epibulbar lesions is excellent.

Pre-cancerous melanosis of the conjunctiva should not be treated unless changes threaten vision. Early intervention can prejudice later treatment, and it is better to observe the condition unless a suspicious biopsy is obtained.

RETINOBLASTOMA

This embryonic tumour of childhood arises in the retina. It accounts for 5 per cent of blindness in children. Histologically, there are sheets of mitotic round cells with areas of calcification and necrosis. Rosettes of neuroblasts may be seen. Rarely there may be differentiation into rods and cones. The tumour eventually spreads through the choroid to the optic nerve and out of the globe.

One-third of the cases have a dominant mode of inheritance. The remainder are sporadic cases, attributed to fresh germinal mutations. The retinal changes are multifocal in origin, and many sporadic cases have lesions in both eyes. In the familial type both eyes are involved in all cases. The tumour may be present at birth but is often not diagnosed until the child is 2 years old. Classically, the lesion calcifies giving a 'cat's eye' white reflex in the eye. Sometimes the diagnosis is only made when secondary strabismus or glaucoma produces symptoms. More advanced lesions cause proptosis.

Treatment

Surgical enucleation is recommended only if the tumour has destroyed over one half of the retina and if the other eye is not involved.

The tumour is radiosensitive. If less than one-third of the fundus is involved, it may be possible to irradiate the lesion and at the same time protect the anterior segment of the eye. Two methods are employed:

As with melanoma, a radon seed tube ring or a Cobalt 60 disc may be sewn on the sclera. A dose of 6000 rads at $\frac{1}{2}$ cm in 1 week is recommended.

Alternatively external irradiation may be used. Small pencil beams about 2·5 cm diameter are directed along nasal and lateral oblique fields avoiding the lens. If a direct beam is required a peephole should be left in the bolus material over the eye. The patient is then encouraged to look into the beam. In this way, radiation build-up may be avoided and some protection provided for the anterior chamber. The recommended dose is 3500 rads in 3 weeks.

Radiotherapy may be combined with an alkylating agent such as cyclophosphamide.

Results

Seventy per cent of patients retain useful vision following irradiation. In recent years the overall 5-year survival, even for bilateral disease, has improved from 25 to 50 per cent. For early disease the survival rate now approaches 100 per cent. The changes in survival patterns have created new problems in genetic counselling.

Complications

Blindness.
Globe atrophy.
Socket contraction.
Scleral ulcer.
Cataract.

One-third of patients treated between 1930 and 1945 developed late radiation-induced malignancy. Now that much smaller doses are being given, the risk has fallen to 1 to 2 per cent.

MISCELLANEOUS EYE TUMOURS

Lymphosarcoma may involve either the lids or the orbit. The lesion is highly radiosensitive and has a better prognosis than lymphosarcoma elsewhere in the body. A dose of 3000 rads in 3 weeks is recommended although it has been stated that a single exposure of 1000 rads to the orbit may be sufficient. There is little information yet on the value of extended field irradiation.

The 5-year survival is 75 per cent.

Reticulum cell sarcoma is a rarer but more serious condition. Most cases rapidly develop generalized disease, in spite of treatment.

Rhabdomyosarcoma is a rare eye lesion. It is moderately radiosensitive and is discussed in Chapter 14. Granulomas may be benign but can sometimes destroy eyesight because of their anatomical position. They often respond to small doses of radiation when other measures have failed. Ectopic salivary tumours of the lacrimal gland are dealt with below.

SALIVARY GLANDS

Eighty per cent of all salivary gland tumours arise in the parotid. This is mainly a serous gland. A further 10 per cent are in the mucous-secreting sub-maxillary and sub-lingual glands. A few cases have been reported in accessory glands in the palate, cheek, tongue and floor of the mouth. Rare cases have also been found in ectopic glands in the nose, trachea and bronchi.

Tumours arise in salivary epithelium and vary from pleomorphic adenomas to highly anaplastic carcinomas. There is no sharp division between benign and malignant disease. In the parotid, on the lip and inside the cheek, these tumours are less likely to be malignant, whereas in the floor of the mouth, on the palate and in the sub-mandibular region the likelihood of malignancy increases.

Salivary gland tumours have been associated with carcinoma of the breast. The reason for this is unknown.

Pathology
Benign.

Mixed parotid: A pleomorphic adenoma of low grade malignancy. This is not really a 'mixed' tumour but the blue staining mucous stroma looks like cartilage and has led to the misnomer.

Muco-epidermoid: Epidermoid areas and mucous-secreting cells. Often seen in parotid, palatal or sub-mandibular glands of children.

Cylindroma or adenoid cystic carcinoma: Usually found in accessory salivary glands, especially the sub-mandibular gland or palate. There are no ducts present. Columns of epithelial cells undergo cystic mucoid change. A curious feature of these tumours is that they spread along nerve sheaths. They may recur up to 25 years later.

Oncocytoma: A very rare, locally malignant tumour of the oxyphil cells.

Adenocarcinoma.

Spheroidal cell carcinoma.

Squamous carcinoma.

Anaplastic carcinoma.

The adenolymphoma or Warthin's papillary cystadenoma is a benign tumour. Recurrence of this tumour after enucleation is merely an expression of the tendency for multiple tumours to occur. Many cases are bilateral.

Clinical Features

Local swelling. Carcinoma grows rapidly and is painful. Contrary to general opinion, however, facial nerve involvement with facial paralysis is not common and appears late.

Treatment

Although needle biopsy has a place in the investigation of some parotid tumours, the modern technique of partial or complete parotidectomy with preservation of the facial nerve has been so well worked out, that most tumours should now be treated by wide excision. Even if the pathology demands the sacrifice of a small length of nerve, it is still possible to perform end-to-end union, and complete recovery of facial movements may be expected.

There is no place for enucleation.

Highly malignant tumours may demand sacrifice of the facial nerve and block dissection of the neck. The cylindroma is particularly aggressive and massive palatal defects are warranted in attempts to resect cylindromas in that area.

Post-operative radiation should be given to all malignant salivary tumours, especially muco-epidermoid lesions and cylindromas. It is of little curative value in highly malignant disease, but prolonged palliation and pain relief is often obtained. Radiotherapy is also reserved for mixed parotid tumours which recur after surgery. This may occur up to 20 years later.

Megavoltage radiation is preferable. A wedge field arrangement is used. A dose of 5500 rads in 5 weeks is recommended. Small fields are usually adequate.

Results

An overall 5-year survival figure is meaningless since mixed parotid tumours, which represent the majority, survive 5 years without treatment. The following figures have been quoted:

Cylindromas   5-year survival = 70 per cent.
Muco-epidermoid   5-year survival = 60 per cent.
Adenocarcinoma   5-year survival = 30 per cent.
Squamous carcinoma   5-year survival = 15 per cent.
Anaplastic   5-year survival = 5 per cent.

Complications

Facial paralysis.

Post-operative fistula. This can be treated with X-ray therapy. A single dose of 400 rads allows the gland to dry up for 6 weeks and facilitates healing.

Frey's syndrome. Red painful sweating cheek due to damage of the auricular temporal division of the trigeminal nerve.

Non-malignant Disease

Mikulicz's disease consists of bilateral painless swellings of the parotid glands associated with a dry mouth, occasionally dry eyes and enlarged lacrimal glands. In the past the disease was confused with tuberculosis, sarcoidosis and other diseases of the parotids. The term is now obsolete, and the disease is associated with an auto-immune condition known as Sjogren's syndrome. This consists of rheumatoid arthritis, xerostomia, xerophthalmia and, rarely, changes in the upper respiratory tract and oesophagus. The treatment is the treatment of the underlying condition. Occasionally, local radiotherapy to the parotid glands may give symptomatic relief. The recommended dose is 1000 rads in 2 weeks.

References

British Medical Journal. Editorial, *Tumours of the Salivary Glands*, 1972, 4 November.
Lancet. *The changing pattern of retinoblastoma*, 1971, 2, 1016.
Maynard, J. *Diseases of the salivary glands*, Hospital Medicine, 1967, April, 619.
Patey, D. *Salivary Tumours*, The Practitioner, 1967, June, 807.

10

Central Nervous System

Nerve tissue is relatively radioresistant in the clinical sense if not in the radiobiological sense. Most brain tumours are derived from the supporting interstitial glial collagen and are called gliomas. Tumours of nerve cells are uncommon.

Gliomas are locally invasive and malignant. They rarely metastasize outside the CNS, possibly because there is no lymph drainage. On the other hand, 30 per cent of all brain tumours are metastatic.

GLIOMAS

The gliomas account for up to 5 per cent of all tumours. Patients usually present with a progressive history of cerebral symptoms such as headaches and confusion. Investigations including arteriogram and brain scan lead to the diagnosis of a space-occupying lesion.

Astrocytoma

These tumours can be divided by their histological appearance into Grades I to IV in ascending degrees of malignancy. The less malignant well-differentiated form contains relatively mature astrocytes with few mitotic figures; it was previously known as the astrocytic glioma or astrocytoma fibrillaire. The more malignant lesions have a pleomorphic appearance with less glial collagen and more hyperchromatic mitotic figures. Unfortunately this highly cellular tumour is more common. It was formerly called spongioblastoma or glioblastoma multiforme.

Grading of astrocytomas requires caution, as neighbouring areas of tumour often have different histological characteristics. Serial biopsy studies suggest that in some neoplasms, transition towards more malignant forms occurs.

The cerebellar astrocytoma of childhood deserves separate attention. It is a well-encapsulated cystic tumour with a low tendency to recurrence after surgical excision.

Oligodendroglioma

This tumour is usually found in the frontal lobe of adults. It consists of gray sheets of 'box'-like cells with little or no stroma. The typical skull X-ray shows flecks of calcium within the tumour.

Ependymoma

This tumour arises from the ependymal cells which line the ventricular walls and the choroid plexus. The tumour, which can be solid or cystic, consists of oval cells that sometimes have a 'pseudo-rosette' appearance. It can also be graded I to IV, the most malignant form being known as ependymoblastoma. A simpler variant, the colloid cyst of the third ventricle, sometimes behaves like a 'ball-cock', producing the clinical picture of intermittent rise in intracranial pressure.

Treatment

Surgery is the treatment of choice for all lesions except medulloblastoma. Complete excision is not always possible. Post-operative supervoltage therapy is recommended for these cases.

The astrocytoma often has occult extension well outside the gross area of tumour involvement. For this reason a generous margin of tissue around the tumour should be treated. The exact dose depends on the volume of tissue irradiated. Recent studies suggest a dose of 4000 rads to the whole brain followed by an additional 2000 rads to the tumour volume.

The ependymoma is moderately radiosensitive, and smaller doses are sometimes adequate. Because of its situation in the ventricle, the ependymoma can cause 'seeding' throughout the sub-arachnoid pathway. If analysis of the spinal fluid yields tumour cells, irradiation of the whole brain and spinal cord is advised.

Results

It is difficult to assess the results of treatment of gliomas, since cases sometimes survive 5 years untreated. However, the following figures have been reported:

Astrocytoma.   Overall 5-year survival = 40 per cent.
Oligodendroglioma.   Overall 5-year survival = 50 per cent.
Ependymoma.   Overall 5-year survival = 40 per cent.

The highly malignant glioblastoma multiforme has a very bad prognosis, although useful palliation of symptoms may sometimes be obtained with radiotherapy. Further palliation may be achieved using 'Epodyl' infusions.

The astrocytoma of childhood has a much better prognosis than the adult form.

MEDULLOBLASTOMA

This embryonic tumour of childhood usually arises in the midline of the cerebellum on the roof of the fourth ventricle. Histologically it consists of small oval 'carrot-shaped' cells. Special staining techniques suggest that the term medulloblastoma includes a number of variants. Failure to recognize this may have led to some confusion in the classification, treatment and prognosis. Medulloblastoma occurs mainly in male children between four and eight years. In adults a rare desmoblastic variety of medulloblastoma is sometimes found. The tumour can seep through the spinal fluid and produce metastasis on the surface of the cord and brain.

Treatment

Surgical removal is rarely possible but fortunately the tumour is radio-sensitive.

It is essential to irradiate the entire brain and spinal cord. Fields should extend to the lower end of the theca which is about 2·5 cm below the second sacral segment. Meticulous care should be taken to ensure that there are no areas left uncovered, such as the base of the frontal lobes.

Supervoltage therapy is recommended. Several techniques have been described (Figure 16).

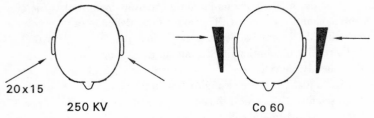

Figure 16   Anterior fields

A posterior field arrangement shaped like a tennis racket is often used (Figure 17). In irradiating the spinal cord through a posterior portal, an inevitable portion of the X-ray beam (the exit dose) passes through the abdominal organs causing nausea. This can be minimized using a short SSD teletherapy unit or electron therapy. In irradiating the skull, care should be taken to protect the eyes.

The recommended dose levels vary widely. A suitable prescription is 3500 rads to the brain in 4 weeks with an additional 1500 rads in 2 weeks to the posterior fossa. The dose to the spinal cord should not exceed 3000 rads. This usually takes a further 4 weeks to deliver. The daily dose should be adjusted to the patient's tolerance. Spinal cord irradiation often results in temporary depression of the bone marrow.

Results

The 5-year survival has increased from 25 to 40 per cent in recent years. Recurrent disease is often noted if the field margins have not been adequately

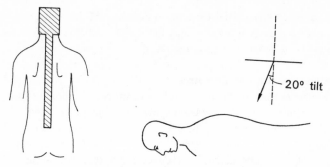

Figure 17   Posterior fields

irradiated. Subsequent growth of the child may be stunted because of vertebral bone damage. Occasionally children develop convulsions later in life due to gliosis and scarring. This is often difficult to differentiate from recurrent disease.

MISCELLANEOUS BRAIN TUMOURS

Unbiopsied Brain Lesions

Tumours of the brain stem and the pineal region of the third ventricle are usually inaccessible even for biopsy.

Surgical decompression when required can be followed by megavoltage radiotherapy. A dose of 5000 rads in 6 to 7 weeks is usually necessary. Five-year survival rates of 25 per cent have been quoted.

The rare tumours of the optic chiasma are usually inoperable. Occasional good results have been quoted following irradiation of these tumours.

Meningioma

This is a benign tumour of the arachnoid cells of the meninges. Most of these lesions can be excised, but radiotherapy may be given if surgery is contra-indicated or if the lesion is inaccessible. Doses of up to 5000 rads are usually necessary.

Acoustic Neuroma

This simple tumour of the vestibular nerve grows very slowly. It lies in the cerebello-pontine angle, and surgical removal is usually possible. Radio-therapy has been tried in a few inoperable cases with variable results.

Chordoma

This tumour arises from embryonic cell rests derived from the foetal notocord. It is found in the vertebrae, sacrococcyx and the basi-sphenoid region of the skull. It is a large soft haemorrhagic tumour that spreads locally in bone and brain. Histologically it consists of characteristic 'physalipherous' cells in a mucoid stroma. Only partial excision is possible. Megavoltage radiotherapy to a dose of 7000 rads in 6 weeks may be tried. The best results are obtained in tumours of the sacrococcygeal region.

Cerebellar Haemangioblastoma

This vascular tumour of the cerebellum was previously thought to be highly malignant. However it has now been shown that 'the name suggests a degree of anaplastic malignancy which the tumour does not remotely possess.' The tumour is certainly radiosensitive and responds to modest doses of radiation between 3000 and 4000 rads in 1 month. The 5-year survival is 76 per cent. Even the 20-year survival is 40 per cent.

Spinal Cord Tumours

Fortunately intra-medullary gliomas are rare. Radiotherapy may be tried, but results are disappointing. However, a combination of surgical decompression and X-ray therapy often results in striking improvement for many years.

Extra-medullary tumours are usually neurofibromas or meningiomas. Both lesions are operable.

Most extra-dural tumours are metastatic.

Metastatic Brain Disease

The primary site should always be sought since the tumour may be sensitive to some specific form of chemotherapy or hormonal therapy, eg, thyroid cancer.

Megavoltage radiotherapy will often relieve metastatic symptoms dramatically. Small doses such as 1600 rads in three treatments to two parallel opposed 12 × 10 cm fields are sufficient. The best results are obtained from metastatic breast carcinoma. Metastatic lung tumours are also worth treating. Stuporous patients occasionally improve sufficiently to return to work for a short time, even though life is not prolonged. Metastatic brain lesions from the prostate or kidney do not respond as well to radiotherapy.

Finally, it is important to recognize that carcinomatous neuropathies may mimic most neurological conditions. These syndromes, which are probably associated with auto-immune mechanisms, may persist even after the primary tumour has been successfully removed.

References

Bouchard, J. *Radiation Therapy of Tumours of the Nervous System*, Lea and Febiger, Philadelphia, 1966.
Buckley, T. F. *Irradiation of cerebral gliomas*, Clin. Radiol., 1969, **20**, 219.
Paterson, E., and Farr, R. F. *Treatment of medulloblastoma*, Acta Radiol., 1953, **39**, 323.

11

Endocrine Glands

PITUITARY TUMOURS

Most pituitary tumours are benign adenomas. Primary carcinoma of the pituitary is rare. Occasionally metastatic deposits lodge in the pituitary fossa and, in the case of widespread breast carcinoma, may bring about a temporary remission by inducing auto-hypophysectomy.

Pathology

Anterior lobe:	Chromophobe adenoma — 60 per cent of cases.
	Eosinophil adenoma — 5 per cent of cases.
	Basophil adenoma — 2 per cent of cases.
Posterior lobe:	Rarely gliomas may involve the floor of the third ventricle and pituitary stalk.
Rathke's pouch:	Craniopharyngioma — 30 per cent of cases. This tumour of young people probably arises in cell rests of the embryonic foregut.

Clinical Features

These can be divided into pressure symptoms and endocrine symptoms.

Pressure symptoms are usually associated with the chromophobe adenoma or the craniopharyngioma. Compression of the optic chiasma causes bitemporal hemianopia. Severe paroxysmal headache suggests raised intracranial pressure, but headache from a purely intrasellar lesion is also recognized. Involvement of the cavernous sinus can produce third nerve palsy with irregular pupils. Cranial nerves IV, V and VI may also be involved. A hypothalamic syndrome featuring obesity, drowsiness, diabetes insipidus and temperature disturbance can occur. Involvement of the uncinate gyrus may cause fits and hallucinations. Decreased libido also occurs.

Endocrine symptoms are associated with both the eosinophilic and chromophobe adenomas. Excessive secretion of growth hormone causes acromegaly in adults, or gigantism in children. Cushing's disease has been associated with the basophilic adenoma and more rarely the chromophobe adenoma. Occasionally these tumours behave in such an aggressive manner that they can be regarded as locally malignant. Excess prolactin may cause galactorrhea.

Hypopituitarism and dwarfism due to destruction of the normal gland often occur with both the chromophobe adenoma and the craniopharyngioma.

Investigations

1 Lateral skull X-ray. This may show a shallow, enlarged or eroded sella turcica. Chromophobe adenomas often have massive asymmetrical suprasellar extensions. Curvilinear calcifications may be seen with the craniopharyngioma.
2 Tomograms and air encephalogram. These may indicate the extent of a suprasellar lesion by showing displacement of the third ventricle and basal cisterns.
3 Visual field perimetry.
4 Hormonal assay: GH, TSH, ACTH, FSH, LH and prolactin.
5 Glucose tolerance test.
6 Metopyrone stimulation test.

Treatment

A combination of radiotherapy and surgery often produces the best result.

Chromophobe adenoma: Radiotherapy alone is recommended for small intrasellar lesions or very large suprasellar tumours where the operative mortality is about 10 per cent. If radiation is used as the initial treatment, surgery may be reserved for patients with rapid loss of vision or where vision fails to improve.

Intracapsular sub-total removal is occasionally advised for chromophobe adenomas with moderate suprasellar extension.

Craniopharyngioma: These lesions are sometimes cystic and may be insensitive to radiation. Surgery is then the treatment of choice. Alternatively, in skilled hands, they can be evacuated and decompressed through the transphenoidal route. Following this the patient can be treated with a radical course of radiation therapy.

Acromegaly: Radiotherapy is recommended for slow-growing intrasellar adenomas with low levels of growth hormone. Stereotactic surgery is best reserved for the more aggressive tumours where a rapid result is desired.

The recommended dose of megavoltage radiation is about 4500 rads in 5 weeks for eosinophil and chromophobe adenomas. Up to 6000 rads in 8 weeks may be required for craniopharyngiomas. Small fields about 4×5 cm are usually adequate. The beam should be directed around a coronal arc centred on the pituitary (Figure 18).

Radioactive isotopes may be implanted, either at open operation or by drilling through the nasal bones in the anterior wall of the pituitary fossa. Gold 198 and yttrium 90 have both been used. Massive doses are required.

Variable results have been claimed for heavy particle accelerators delivering single doses of up to 4000 rads. However, these machines are costly and are not readily available for clinical work.

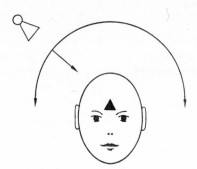

Figure 18   Coronal arc for pituitary irradiation

Cryosurgery and radiofrequency heat coagulation have also been used, but these techniques are still experimental.

Results

Up to 90 per cent cure rates are claimed for chromophobe tumours. The full effects of treatment should not be assessed until one year has elapsed.

The treatment of acromegaly is less satisfactory, but visual defects usually improve and headache is often relieved. The disease process may be retarded, but systemic effects on the cardiovascular system and carbohydrate metabolism are often unaltered for several years. Results are best judged by changes in the glucose tolerance test or reduction in the level of growth hormone. Untreated acromegalics rarely survive beyond 60 years of age.

Variable results have been reported with cystic craniopharyngiomas, and further trials are under way. The non-cystic variety responds to radiation.

The results of pituitary irradiation may be interpreted in the light of recent radiobiological experiments. Immediate cell death occurs only after enormous doses of radiation. At conventional dose levels, cells are damaged but remain functionally active until the subsequent mitosis which, in the case of the pituitary, may not be due for many years. This explains why radiation is more effective in controlling the pressure symptoms associated with expanding pituitary adenomas, than in controlling the functional endocrine features of acromegaly.

Complications

Hypopituitarism may develop after several years. Cortisone, thyroid and sex hormone replacement therapy are indicated.

Sudden haemorrhage into the tumour can cause blindness.

Pituitary implantation by the transphenoidal route carries the risk of meningitis, cerebrospinal rhinorrhoea, blindness, third nerve palsy and diabetes insipidus.

THYROID CARCINOMA

This rare disease usually arises in a previously abnormal thyroid gland. The condition is commoner in areas where goitre is endemic, such as Switzerland where it accounts for 3·5 per cent of all cancer deaths. The main aetiological factors seem to be increased secretion of TSH and exposure of the growing gland to ionizing radiation. However, radioactive iodine treatment of thyrotoxicosis has not been implicated. Thyroid diseases are more common in women, but this preponderance is not so marked with differentiated carcinoma.

Random autopsy studies suggest that asymptomatic occult islands of thyroid cancer exist in the thyroid glands of 5 per cent of elderly patients. The disease is similar in this respect to cancer of the prostate.

Classification

1. PAPILLARY. This slow-growing tumour occurs in children and young adults. It consists of fibrous stalks covered with atypical epithelial cells. Metastatic spread is to the regional lymph nodes where it may lie dormant for years.

2. FOLLICULAR. This somewhat rarer tumour is also slow growing. It is found in the age group 30 to 50 years. The lesion partly resembles normal thyroid tissue with columnar epithelium and variable acinar formation which frequently contains colloid. Blood spread is common.

Follicular carcinoma can be sub-divided into two distinct groups on clinical and histological grounds. In one group the tumour is confined to its capsule and is easily removed. In the other, the lesion is more anaplastic and often presents with metastatic disease.

It has been noted that follicular tumours with papillary elements behave like papillary tumours, even though the bulk of tumour tissue is follicular.

3. MEDULLARY. This is an extremely rare solid tumour of the parafollicular 'C' cells. Most of these tumours secrete calcitonin. The tumour has been associated with a familial neurocutaneous syndrome characterized by multiple mucosal neuromas and also with phaeochromocytoma.

4. UNDIFFERENTIATED. This anaplastic tumour is one of the most aggressive known. Typically it occurs in the over-60 age group.

Clinical Features

The differentiation from simple goitre is difficult in the early stages, and an average delay of 1 year occurs before diagnosis has been noted. There may be a history of rapid glandular enlargement. On examination the swelling is often fixed to surrounding tissues. Hardness is a poor sign of malignancy. Hoarseness accompanying thyroid enlargement is often associated with thyroid cancer and usually indicates recurrent laryngeal nerve involvement. However, hoarseness is not pathognomonic of cancer since it is also found in sub-acute thyroiditis.

Investigations

X-ray examination is necessary to show the extent of the disease and to exclude lung metastases. Calcification is sometimes seen in papillary and medullary carcinomas.

Radioactive iodine scans may reveal 'cold' nodules which are often the site of carcinoma; 'hot' nodules are never malignant. Following thyroid ablation, tracer studies may detect functioning metastases.

The diagnosis can be confirmed by drill biopsy, especially if an anaplastic lesion is suspected. The danger of spreading the tumour by this investigation has probably been exaggerated.

Treatment

The treatment of each pathological variety will be considered in turn. The place of surgery is controversial and the best therapeutic combinations have yet to be established. Meanwhile many clinicians manage thyroid carcinoma in the following ways:

PAPILLARY. Surgical excision with removal of involved nodes is recommended. Occasionally lobectomy is adequate for a solitary nodule. This should be supplemented by full thyroid hormone replacement therapy in an attempt to suppress pituitary drive. Metastatic disease may occasionally respond to radioactive iodine therapy.

FOLLICULAR. Total thyroidectomy. In the absence of metastatic disease, thyroid replacement should follow. If tracer studies reveal functioning metastases, these may be treated by radio-iodine ablation. This procedure may be repeated at intervals, so long as the dose of whole body radiation does not exceed 400 rads. Pulmonary fibrosis and aplastic anaemia are recognized hazards of radio-iodine therapy. There has been a suggestion that these risks can be reduced by using I^{124} which gives a better radiation dose distribution to the gland. Aggressive disease can sometimes be suppressed by large doses of thyroxine. The unwanted peripheral effects of thyroid hormone can then be blocked with propranolol and guanethedine.

MEDULLARY. *Surgery.* Residual disease may sometimes respond to large doses of radiotherapy. Up to 5500 rads in 5 weeks are required. Radio-iodine-therapy and thyroid hormone suppression are of no value.

ANAPLASTIC. *Radiotherapy.* Supervoltage radiation to a dose of 4500 rads in 4 weeks. Fields should be designed to protect the cervical cord. These tumours never take up radioactive iodine and are not suppressed by thyroid hormone.

SPINAL METASTASES. Differentiated thyroid carcinoma often spreads exclusively to bone, and vertebral collapse may lead to paraplegia. This is a surgical emergency and necessitates urgent laminectomy and cord decompression. This should be followed by I[131] therapy, local radiation and diuretic therapy. Treatment may be effective even up to two months after the onset of paraplegia.

Results

Differentiated carcinoma is compatible with long life. Indeed it was formerly called benign metastasizing thyroid carcinoma. One long-term follow-up series of papillary lesions has shown a prognosis slightly better than that of the general population! The results with follicular and medullary lesions are also good, if not quite so spectacular.

Anaplastic carcinoma is often radiosensitive. However, the tumour recurs rapidly, and the 5-year survival rate is less than 10 per cent. The prognosis worsens with age.

PANCREAS AND ADRENAL

Carcinoma of the pancreas is a depressing disease with a gloomy prognosis. There is little place for radiotherapy in the management of this condition.

Islet-cell tumours of the pancreas belong to a spectrum of peptide-secreting adenomas. The insulin-producing group (beta cell tumours) are benign, but the Zollinger-Ellison syndrome may be associated with a lesion that metastasizes slowly to the liver. Pancreatic irradiation is not indicated, but an occasional attempt may be made to suppress excessive gastric secretion by radiotherapy.

Radiotherapy is usually not required for tumours of the adrenal cortex. This is also true for most cases of phaeochromocytoma. However, 11 per cent of medullary tumours of the adrenal gland are malignant, and these patients may develop functioning metastases requiring palliative radiation.

Neuroblastoma of the adrenal is highly radiosensitive. The treatment of this tumour is discussed in Chapter 21. The primary treatment of ganglioneuroma is surgery.

It is convenient to include ectopic pineloma here. This rare tumour may present with precocious puberty, diabetes insipidus, hypopituitarism or visual disturbance. Some reports suggest that a combination of surgery and radiotherapy gives the best result.

References

British Medical Journal. Editorial, *Craniopharyngomas*, 1972, March, 764.
British Journal of Radiology. Thyroid Cancer Symposium, 1971, October, 819.
Connolly, R. C. *The Pituitary Adenomas*, Brit. J. Med., 1969, 2, 1706.
Kramer, S. *The Treatment of Pituitary Adenomas*, Canadian Med. Assoc. J., 1968, 1120.
Memorial Sloan-Kettering Cancer Bulletin. *Thyroid Carcinoma*, 1972, Vol 2, 1.

12

Thorax

LUNG CANCER

The main aetiological factors in this disease are well known. They include cigarette smoking, atmospheric pollution and asbestosis. Since 1957 the disease has been increasing in all groups of the population except the medical profession where it has been declining. There seems little doubt that this is due to decreased smoking habits among doctors.

Clinical Features

Patients may present with chest symptoms such as cough, haemoptysis, dyspnoea, pain and dysphagia. They may also present with pneumonia or superior vena caval obstruction. Other clinical features include malaise, anorexia, loss of weight and finger clubbing. Metastatic symptoms may occur due to deposits in bone, brain, liver and elsewhere. Non-metastatic syndromes involving the endocrine system, nervous system and skin are well recognized.

Investigations

1 Chest X-ray.
2 Bronchoscopy — bronchoscopic washings for cytology.
3 Sputum for cytology. An aerosol may be used to make the patient cough.
4 Gland biopsy.
5 Mediastinoscopy.
6 Needle biopsy.

Histology

Squamous cell carcinoma — 40 per cent.

Anaplastic carcinoma — 45 per cent. This group is divided into a large cell type and a small cell type ('oat'-cell). Mixed cell types are often seen.

Adenocarcinoma is relatively more common in women.

Rare tumours include bronchiolar alveolar cell carcinoma and argentaffinoma.

Treatment

Surgery is the treatment of choice for squamous cell carcinoma. If the tumour appears operable, a thoracotomy is advised followed by lobectomy or pneumonectomy if possible.

The following criteria usually mean the tumour is inoperable:

1. Widening of the carina due to glands in the angle.
2. Both lungs involved.
3. Blood-stained pleural effusion.
4. Hoarseness due to laryngeal nerve involvement.
5. Phrenic nerve paralysis.
6. Metastases.

The place of pre-operative radiotherapy in squamous carcinoma is currently being investigated in several centres. It has been suggested that radiation can render some inoperable lesions amenable to surgery.

Radiation therapy is the treatment of choice for oat-cell carcinoma even if the disease appears operable. Most growths arise within 2-3 cm from the carina and usually involve the peribronchial and mediastinal glands. An adequate margin around the tumour should be treated. Megavoltage radiation is advised. A dose of 4500 rads in 3 to 4 weeks, depending upon field size, is usually sufficient to control local disease. Higher doses do not seem to improve cure rates but they do lead to increased pulmonary fibrosis.

The palliative value of radiation is considerable, but palliation should be reserved for those patients with symptoms to palliate. Modest doses of about 3000 rads in 2 weeks are sufficient to alleviate:

1. Pain due to chest wall invasion.
2. Dyspnoea.
3. Superior vena caval obstruction.
4. Haemoptysis.
5. Dysphagia.
6. Pain due to Pancoast's syndrome.

Small metastatic deposits in the skin can be treated with single exposures of 1500 rads. Bony deposits also respond to palliative doses of radiation. Brain metastasis can often be controlled with short courses of therapy. A dose of 2000 rads in five treatments is well tolerated.

Pleural effusions can be controlled with installation of nitrogen mustard. A dose of 0·5 milligrams per kilogram is recommended. Good palliative responses have been obtained using cyclophosphamide in oat-cell carcinoma, but no cures have been reported.

Results

The prognosis in this disease is gloomy with an overall 5-year survival rate of less than 10 per cent. In the highly selected group of operable squamous cell carcinomas of the lung the 5-year survival rate is 30 per cent. The survival rate for early oat-cell carcinoma is under 5 per cent. A few inoperable tumours may occasionally be saved by radical radiation therapy.

Palliative radiotherapy plays an important role. Although patients do not live longer, distressing symptoms are often relieved and bedridden patients are occasionally made sufficiently ambulant to return to work.

OESOPHAGUS

Aetiology

Carcinoma of the oesophagus has a high incidence in Bantus who drink native beer brewed in metal drums. It has also been described in maize eaters. The disease is relatively common in Japan and may be related to drinking hot saki and eating spices. A curious connection has been reported between oesophageal cancer and molybdenum deficiency in gardens. Excessive smoking and alcohol intake have also been blamed. In Britain many cases in women are associated with the Plummer-Vinson syndrome.

Pathology

The tumour arises at points of anatomical narrowing. The upper third is the supra-aortic part. The middle third is that part related to the aortic arch and left main bronchus. The lower third is related to the stomach. Fifteen per cent of tumours arise in the upper third; these are mainly in women. Thirty-five per cent occur in the middle third; males predominate in this region. The remaining 50 per cent are in the lower third.

Most tumours are squamous cell carcinomas with varying degrees of differentiation. A few adenocarcinomas and sarcomas have been described. Even basal cell carcinoma has been reported.

More than one-third of patients are incurable when first seen. These patients have evidence of blood-borne metastases, lymphatic spread remote from the primary tumour, oesophago-tracheal fistula or a primary tumour longer than 10 cm. In Bantu natives many patients are seen with total involvement of the oesophagus.

Clinical Features

Anorexia and loss of weight.
Dysphagia.
Sub-sternal discomfort.
Regurgitation.
Vomiting.
Laryngeal nerve paralysis.

Investigations
> Chest X-ray.
> Barium swallow.
> Oesophagoscopy.
> Biopsy.

Treatment

SURGERY. Generally speaking, surgery is preferred for lesions of the lower third and radiotherapy for those higher up. In Edinburgh, radiation has been recommended for all cases, whatever the level. Resection with oesophago-gastrostomy should only be attempted if the surgeon feels he has a reasonable chance of curing the patient. If at operation he finds the tumour is inoperable, a simple by-pass procedure is recommended.

Palliative thoracotomy carries a high mortality, and simpler means of relief are available. Formerly Souttar's tube was used to relieve obstruction. It only takes a few minutes to pass. However, the tube is made of metal, and a number of perforations have been reported. It is now outmoded by plastic tubes such as Mousseau-Barbin and Celestin. These are usually positioned through a gastrostomy from below.

RADIOTHERAPY. Rotation or multiple field megavoltage therapy is recommended for tumours of the middle and upper third. An estimate of the length of the growth should be made — tumours often measure 5 cm — and an adequate margin allowed. It is worth spending some time with these patients since careful attention to detail can double the curability of the disease. Accurate localization is essential. The posture of the patient during treatment should be simulated in the planning room beforehand. The best dose distribution is obtained with rotation therapy, especially in the thoracic oesophagus. The most frequently treated volume is an ellipsoidal or cylindrical solid of rotation 14×7 cm. In thoraco-cervical tumours the patient's shoulders are a geometrical obstacle to good dosimetry; conical therapy with a wedge filter provides a sophisticated answer to this problem (Figure 19). The recommended dose is 5000 rads in 4 weeks.

Various other radiotherapeutic procedures have been tried. These include intracavitary radium or radioactive tantalum suspended in a Souttar's tube. Direct gold seed implants have also been used.

Results

Five-year survival = 20 per cent.

Results are slightly better for the higher lesions. Smaller doses of radiation often give palliative relief of distressing symptoms. Radiation has the additional advantages of leaving the patient with a normal voice and a normal stomach.

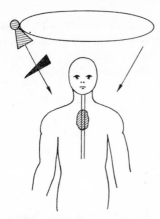

Figure 19   Conical wedge therapy

The best results with carcinoma of the oesophagus have been obtained by Nakayama and co-workers in Japan. They recommend an aggressive combination of radiotherapy and surgery. Unfortunately, the Japanese results have not been repeated elsewhere.

TRACHEA

Tumours of the trachea are extremely rare and are often inoperable. Radio-therapy has provided prolonged control in a few cases.

THYMUS

The thymus is the immunological centre in early life. Here thymic hormone 'instructs' stem cells to become thymic lymphocytes. These then migrate out and are immunologically competent in later life. In the neonatal inductive phase, infants acquire immunological tolerance to their own antigens; that is, they learn to differentiate between 'self' and 'non-self'. In adult life, alteration of this immune apparatus may provoke auto-immune disease.

Thus the large thymic shadow seen on X-ray in children is a normal structure. In the past many of these children were mistakenly treated with radiation; unfortunately a number subsequently developed thyroid carcinoma. In adults, however, a hyperplastic thymus gland may be associated with a thymic tumour or with auto-immune disease, especially myasthenia gravis.

Seventy-five per cent of patients with thymic tumours have myasthenia gravis but only 15 per cent of patients with myasthenia have thymic tumours. Only those patients with thymic enlargement should be treated with radiation.

Thymic Tumour

This rare tumour is the most common swelling in the anterior mediastinum.

D

HISTOLOGY. Mixed cell thymo-lymphoepithelioma. Cells may be predominantly lymphocytic resembling Hodgkin's disease, or predominantly epithelial producing Hassell's corpuscles.

A few cases of lymphosarcoma, Hodgkin's disease and teratoma have also been described.

CLINICAL FEATURES
   Myasthenia gravis.
   Dyspnoea.
   Cough and stridor.
   Superior vena caval obstruction.
   Phrenic nerve irritation.

INVESTIGATIONS. Straight and lateral chest X-rays. If these are negative, pneumography is indicated. This involves injection of carbon dioxide into the mediastinum. The technique may uncover a tumour just anterior to the aorta where it merges with the pericardium.

TREATMENT. A combination of surgery and radiotherapy is indicated because the tumour is often locally malignant. A dose of up to 4500 rads in 4 weeks is recommended. In those cases with myasthenia, part of the radiation should be given pre-operatively, otherwise the myasthenia worsens during the post-operative period. The reason for this is unknown. The recommended pre-operative dose is 2500 rads in 2 to 3 weeks. If at operation the tumour is found to be invasive, a course of post-operative radiation to an additional 2500 rads is advised.

RESULTS. Malignant lymphomas of the thymus do relatively well with a 5-year survival of over 50 per cent. Epithelial tumours have a poorer prognosis. Myasthenia gravis does not improve with radiation therapy.

COMPLICATIONS. The main complications of X-ray therapy are a worsening of the myasthenia, retrosternal pain, pulmonary infection and fibrosis. Myasthenia is controlled by an anti-cholinergic drug such as neostigmine. The dose of neostigmine is the maximum the patient will tolerate, but caution should be used since drug overdosage may lead to a cholinergic crisis. This produces muscle weakness which may be difficult to distinguish from a myasthenic crisis.

References

Deeley, T. J. *Treatment of carcinoma of the bronchus*, Brit. J. Radiol., 1967, **40**, 801.
Medical Research Council Report. *Radiotherapy of oat-celled carcinoma of the Bronchus*, Lancet, 1969, **2**, 501.
Nakayama, K. *Pre-operative irradiation in the treatment of carcinoma of the oesophagus*, Clin. Radiol., 1964, **15**, 232.
Pearson, J. G. *Radiotherapy in Oesophageal Carcinoma*, Am. J. Roent., 1969, **105**, 500.

13

Abdomen

Malignant disease of the gastro-intestinal tract is mainly the province of surgery. There are several reasons for this. Most of the lesions are adeno-carcinomas and are relatively radioresistant. It is also difficult to know the full extent of the tumour prior to laparotomy. Added to this, abdominal irradiation is poorly tolerated. Nevertheless, in a few cases, where patients were unfit for surgery, an occasional radiotherapeutic cure has been reported.

The prognosis in cancer of the alimentary tract improves as one descends from the oesophagus to the colon. Until recently the role of radiotherapy has been mainly palliative, but there is now an increased interest in combining radiotherapy with surgery in the hope of improving prognosis at various sites. In some studies, treatment is being combined with a chemotherapeutic agent, such as 5-fluorouracil.

Radiation is the treatment of choice, of course, in the rare abdominal lymphomas. These may be confined to the stomach in some cases, but even where there is widespread dissemination, the disease can often be controlled by radiotherapy for long periods of time.

A few of the more important features at each site are briefly outlined below.

CARCINOMA OF THE STOMACH

This disease accounts for about 10 per cent of cancer deaths in western countries. It is found in lower socioeconomic groups, especially in Japan, and may be associated with dietary habits.

Surgery is the treatment of choice, the extent of the operation depending upon the extent of the disease. Unfortunately, most cases have metastases, especially in the liver, and the 5-year survival is only 10 per cent. Radiotherapy does not improve prognosis.

SMALL BOWEL CANCER

Malignant tumours of the small intestine are relatively rare. Again the primary treatment is surgical, but it is important to exclude lymphomas which account for one-third of all cases.

In those patients with lymphomas the treatment technique depends on the extent of the disease. For large volumes, a moving strip method is usually recommended. The dose varies between 2000 and 3000 rads depending on the grade and stage of the disease. It is important to shield the kidneys when the dose exceeds 2000 rads in 2 weeks.

The prognosis for abdominal lymphomas is relatively good in the short term but long-term results are variable (see also Chapter 15).

LARGE BOWEL CANCER

Carcinoma of the lower alimentary tract is about three times as common as gastric carcinoma. Some cases are associated with familial polyposis and ulcerative colitis, but in the majority of cases the aetiological factors are unknown. About 50 per cent of cases occur in the rectum, and the remainder are distributed throughout the colon.

The principles of surgical treatment are outlined in the standard textbooks. In carcinoma of the rectum, the cure rate following surgery alone is 50 per cent. Ten per cent of cases recur locally in the pelvis. These are mostly tumours of the lower rectum with high-grade malignancy and lymph spread. Combined radiation and surgery has been recommended for these high risk cases. Radical radiation may be given to patients who are unfit for surgery or who refuse operation. Doses of up to 6000 rads in 6 weeks have been given on megavoltage therapy. In a few small series, survival results equalling those of surgery have been reported.

Recently pre-operative radiation has been recommended for all cases. Fields should include the entire pelvis and extend up to the second lumbar vertebra. Doses of 4500 to 5000 rads in 5 weeks have been given. It is claimed that survival is increased and local recurrence eliminated.

Excellent palliative results have been obtained in the treatment of local perineal recurrence. In most cases, pain can be relieved and haemorrhage controlled. The recommended palliative dose is about 4000 rads in 3 to 4 weeks.

PANCREAS AND LIVER

Carcinoma involving these organs carries a dismal prognosis. Radiation adds little to survival. Even palliative results are disappointing.

Recent work suggests that it may be worth treating some cases of Hodgkin's disease involving the liver, but the full results of these trials are not yet available.

CARCINOMA OF THE ANUS

The indications for radiotherapy in anal cancer were carefully studied several years ago, and for this reason the disease is discussed in a little more detail.

Classification

Tumours of the anus can be divided into those involving the anal margin and those involving the anal canal. Anal margin tumours are commoner in men. Canal tumours are commoner in women. The anal canal measures about 4 cm long. The lower canal has a rich nerve supply, and lesions in this region are often extremely painful.

Tumours of the anus may be ulcerative, nodular or proliferative. In the margin they are often well-differentiated squamous cell lesions with keratin formation. Rarely a basal cell carcinoma may be seen. In the canal there is less keratin, and transitional epithelium may merge with columnar epithelium of the rectum. Tumours may arise in an old sinus. Occasionally adeno-carcinoma of the distal rectum may present at the anus.

Treatment

SURGERY. Tumours of the margin require wide local excision using diathermy. If the anorectal ring is removed, incontinence results. Tumours lying in the canal require abdominal-perineal excision of the rectum.

It is important to remember that the anal margin drains directly to the inguinal nodes whereas the anal canal drains along the haemorrhoidal vessels. This can influence the extent of surgical dissection when nodes are involved.

RADIOTHERAPY. Radiation is best reserved for small growths and for advanced disease. This has the advantage of lower morbidity in selected patients. Small, well-differentiated localized lesions on the verge and low canal can be treated by a radium implant. This preserves sphincter control. A flat plaque-like lesion limited to one side may be treated by a single plane implant. Larger tumours require a cylindrical implant. The recommended dose is 5500 rads in 7 days. 'Indian Club' radium needles, preferentially loaded at one end, may be used to build up the dose at the inner end of the implant. An additional layer of needles can be crossed at right angles, at the outer end of the implant in buttock skin.

Medium-sized tumours should be treated surgically. If, however, surgery is contra-indicated for any reason, megavoltage therapy may be used. A dose of up to 5500 rads in 4 to 5 weeks is recommended. Very advanced lesions may be treated palliatively with somewhat smaller doses. Occasionally a defunctioning colostomy is necessary.

Results

Overall 5-year survival rate = 35 per cent.

Localized tumours of the margin do well. The prognosis deteriorates with nodal involvement.

In experienced hands morbidity is low, but the perineum has a relatively low tolerance to radiation and indiscriminate treatment can cause necrosis, incontinence or anal stricture.

References

Allen, C. V., and Fletcher, W. S. *Pre-operative Irradiation of Rectosigmoid Carcinoma*, Am. J. Roent., 1972, **114**, 504.

Leeming, R. H., Stearns, M. W., and Deddish, M. R. *Pre-operative irradiation in Rectal Carcinoma*, Radiol., 1961, **77**, 257.

Williams, I. G. *Carcinoma of the anus and anal canal*, Clin. Radiol., 1962, **13**, 30.

14

Bone and Soft Tissues

OSTEOSARCOMA

Most cases occur in young people in their late teens. In older patients the tumour is usually associated with Paget's disease.

Sites
Seventy-five per cent arise in the metaphysis of long bones near the knee joint.

Histology
A pleomorphic tumour with multinucleate giant cells and spindle cells in a matrix of cartilage, fibrous and osteoid tissue. The diagnostic criterion is the formation of bone and osteoid tissue by tumour cells.

There are five types:

1 Osteoblastic.
2 Chondroblastic.
3 Fibroblastic.
4 Mixed.
5 Anaplastic.

Spread
Bloodstream to lungs. Chest X-ray should be obtained before treatment.

Clinical Features
A painful lump with dysfunction.

X-ray Appearance
1 Bone destruction and bone formation producing osteolytic or osteoblastic lesions.
2 Codman's triangle. (Cortical erosion with undermining of edges.)
3 Sun-ray spiculation.
4 Onion-peel layers.
5 Periosteal reaction.

Biopsy

Open biopsy is preferred since it produces less tension and less risk of dissemination. Drill or punch biopsy is sometimes recommended after radiotherapy has been started.

Treatment

The place of amputation is controversial and the relative role of surgery and radiotherapy must await controlled trials. Meanwhile the following regimen is recommended:

1. Radiotherapy. Megavoltage radiation using parallel opposed fields. Dose up to 8000 rads in 8 weeks.
2. Review after 8 months. If there is evidence of active disease and the chest X-ray remains clear, amputation above the proximal joint is recommended. The delay avoids unnecessary initial amputation by allowing occult lung metastases time to develop.
3. A solitary lung metastases occurring after 5 years may sometimes be successfully removed by lobectomy.
4. Citrovorum rescue chemotherapy (see Chapter 24).

Results

The 5-year survival is 20 per cent. The prognosis is best in low-grade osteoblastic tumours in young patients. Even if the lesion is not cured, radiotherapy often relieves pain, and the swelling may disappear. Later, osteolytic lesions may recalcify and pathological fractures may heal.

Excellent results from surgery alone are obtained in the very rare parosteal osteosarcoma.

Complications

Late radiation effects can cause muscle atrophy, disability and deformity.

CHONDROSARCOMA

This tumour is usually found in middle-aged persons. It does not respond well to radiotherapy. Treatment is amputation. The 5-year survival is 40 per cent. The prognosis is better in the long bones than in the axial skeleton.

ROUND CELL SARCOMA

Round cell sarcoma is an inexact term that includes primary reticulum cell sarcoma of bone, Ewing's tumour and neuroblastoma.

Reticulum Cell Sarcoma of Bone

This solitary tumour of bone is derived from the reticulum cells in the bone marrow. The lesion is identical to reticulum cell sarcoma in lymph nodes. Lymph node metastases occur more frequently than in other primary bone tumours. The tumour is radiosensitive, and the 5-year survival rate is 50 per cent. Amputation is reserved for recurrence. A fuller discussion is given under lymphomas.

Ewing's Tumour and Neuroblastoma

Some authors believe these lesions to be the same. However, a number of different features can be recognized. On histological examination both neoplasms show small round cells with dark nuclei and a little clear cytoplasm. The neuroblastoma may also have rosette clusters, eosinophilic fibrils and maturation to neurones with calcification. Other differences are outlined in Table X.

TABLE X

Comparison of Ewing's tumour and neuroblastoma

	Ewing's tumour	**Neuroblastoma**
Age	Teenagers	Infants and young children
Spread	Lungs, long bones	Skull, lymph nodes, liver
Investigations	X-ray appearance of 'onion-peel' periosteal new bone	Urinary catecholamines
5-year survival	15 per cent	35 per cent; better in infants

Both lesions are highly radiosensitive, although high dosage (5000 rads in 5 weeks) has been recommended for Ewing's tumour. The entire medullary canal of involved bone should be treated. A trial is under way to test the effectiveness of whole body radiation in this disease. Because of the high incidence of disseminated disease in both conditions, radiation should be combined with chemotherapy. Initial results of trials are encouraging. Neuroblastoma is discussed further under paediatric tumours (Chapter 21).

OSTEOCLASTOMA

Some clinicians prefer to call this Giant Cell Tumour of Bone since it may not arise from the osteoclasts.

Incidence

The disease is more common in young women.

Sites

It occurs most often in the epiphysis of long bones near the knee joint and also in the clavicle and patella.

Pathology
Osteoclastoma is usually benign but it can become locally aggressive with extension to soft tissue and articular cartilage. Ten per cent are either initially malignant or undergo sarcomatous degeneration.

Histology
Multinucleate giant cells are seen with up to 250 nuclei! The stroma consists of mitosing mononuclear spindle cells. If there is an excess of bone, cartilage or fibrous tissue present then the lesion is not an osteoclastoma but a variant.

The malignant form of the disease merges with osteogenic sarcoma.

X-ray Appearance
Characteristic but not pathognomonic. Eccentric cystic rarefaction involving both the epiphysis and metaphysis gives a 'soap bubble' appearance.

Differential Diagnosis
Giant cell variants include:

1   Hyperparathyroidism.
2   Aneurysmal bone cyst.
3   Reparative granuloma of the jaw.
4   Non-ossifying fibroma.
5   Traumatized solitary bone cyst.

Treatment
1   Excision with removal of surrounding shell of normal bone followed by bone graft.
2   Curettage is poor treatment since it is followed by 50 per cent recurrence.
3   Megavoltage radiotherapy:
    a   Where surgery is contra-indicated.
    b   Recurrence after surgery where amputation is refused.
    c   Unusual site, eg, vertebra.
    d   Sarcomatous degeneration. As for osteogenic sarcoma.

A dose of 4000 rads in 4 weeks is adequate to control most cases of osteoclastoma. Malignant disease requires higher doses.

Results
Five-year survival = 80 per cent. Note that following radiotherapy there is a temporary 'osteolytic thrust' with osteolysis and enlargement.

Complications
Late radiation damage to bone and joint causing disability and deformity.

BONE METASTASES

The commonest bone tumour is a metastatic tumour. It may arise from any primary site, but the following midline structures are usually mentioned:

1   Thyroid.
2   Breast.
3   Lung.
4   Kidney.
5   Prostate.

Secondary deposits are rarely found below the knee or elbow except from the thyroid or kidney. Both these tumours often produce massive bone destruction with pulsating metastases. A solitary deposit in the humerus is frequently from a hypernephroma.

Treatment

The management may be remembered under the five P's.

1. PRIMARY. This should always be sought since the disease may respond to specific hormonal or chemotherapy.

2. PALLIATE. Treatment is always palliative and radical therapy is not indicated.

3. PAIN. Radiotherapy often gives dramatic relief. Generally the therapist should direct the fields to include the painful region as well as the area of radiographic involvement. The dose level is usually about 60 to 70 per cent of a radical therapeutic dose. This varies between 1500 rads in two treatments for small fields to 3000 rads in 2 weeks for larger fields. The exact dose depends on the radiosensitivity of the tumour and on patient response.

4. PATHOLOGICAL FRACTURE. A fracture of the lower limb should be treated by open reduction, particularly those in the shaft of femur where a nail may be used, and neck of femur where a prosthesis may be possible. This should be followed by irradiation. Elsewhere radiotherapy may promote bony union without surgery. Occasionally pathological fractures heal spontaneously.

5. PARAPLEGIA. Sudden vertebral collapse is an emergency situation necessitating immediate surgical decompression followed by radiotherapy together with cytoxic and diuretic therapy. This is particularly important in diseases with an otherwise good prognosis such as Hodgkin's disease or thyroid carcinoma.

SOFT TISSUE TUMOURS

These tumours can occur at any anatomical site in the body. They are especially common in the extremities.

If possible they should be classified by tissue of origin; eg, fibrosarcoma, liposarcoma, rhabdomyosarcoma, etc.

If this is not possible then a simple classification can be used; eg, differentiated sarcoma, poorly differentiated sarcoma, undifferentiated sarcoma.

Soft tissue sarcomas usually spread via lymph nodes in the first instance, followed by blood-borne metastases.

Diagnosis

Any enlarging sub-cutaneous tumour of recent origin should be regarded as malignant until proved otherwise. Biopsy is mandatory. X-rays are necessary to determine whether there is bone involvement or lung metastases.

Treatment

1 Wide excision (no enucleation).
2 Radical radiotherapy 2 weeks later.
3 Radiotherapy alone if there is (*a*) bone fixation; (*b*) bone destruction; (*c*) mutilation.

Megavoltage. Dose up to 7000 rads in 7 weeks. This can be followed by a policy of observation or amputation if necessary.

Note that many of these slow-growing tumours were formerly thought to be radioresistant because they were unchanged 6 months after radiation treatment. Nevertheless they often heal eventually.

Fibrosarcoma

Seventy-five per cent of soft tissue tumours. The lesion can arise in soft tissue or in the outer layer of periosteum of bone. The borderline between fibroma and fibrosarcoma is not clear, and growth is often slow. If a benign fibroma is locally excised and recurs, it should be treated as malignant.

Five-year survival = 50 per cent.

Poorly Differentiated Sarcoma

This is the second largest group of soft tissue neoplasms. The lesion is often radiosensitive but may not be radiocurable.

Neuro-fibrosarcoma

Often found in supraclavicular region, the disease is extremely painful and radioresistant.

Synovial Sarcoma

This condition may occur in the leg or knee joint of young adults. Local excision plus radiation is recommended. Amputation is rarely justified since nothing controls the really malignant tumour and less aggressive lesions respond to radiation.

Five-year survival = 40 per cent.

Liposarcoma

It is doubtful if the simple lipoma ever becomes a malignant liposarcoma. Most cases are probably lipo-fibrosarcomas and should be treated as fibrosarcomas.

Five-year survival = 20 per cent.

Kaposi's Sarcoma

See Chapter 6.

Dermatofibrosarcoma

This is often a slow-growing localized skin mass. It is usually locally recurrent and radioresistant.

Rhabdomyosarcoma

In adults this disease is mainly found in the nasopharynx but it may also occur in the palate, orbit, antrum, nasal fossa and middle ear. It is divided into the following types:

1 Pleomorphic — adults.
2 Alveolar — adolescent.
3 Embryonal (often no muscle fibres) — child.
4 Sarcoma botryoides. A grape-like tumour related to mucous membrane in the female urogenital tract and the vaginal walls. Also found in the male urogenital sinus.

These tumours are radiosensitive although only rarely radiocurable. A dose of 5000 rads in 5 weeks is often adequate to control local disease. Actinomycin D has also been recommended. Surgery can be used to restore the airway in adults with head and neck lesions, but most cases have early distant metastases.

Overall 5-year survival = 20 per cent.

Lymphangiosarcoma

This rare multi-nodular haemorrhagic tumour may develop in lymphoedematous limbs. This can occur following radical mastectomy for carcinoma of the breast. The disease is totally radioresistant.

Angiosarcoma

This lesion is also rare and difficult to diagnose. It should not be confused with the simple hamartoma. The tumour often responds to moderate doses of radiation.

References

Cade, S. *Osteogenic Sarcoma*, J. R. Coll. Surg. Edin., 1965, **1**, 111.

Johnson, R. E., and Pomeroy, T. C. *Ewing's Sarcoma*, Am. J. Roent., 1972, **114**, 532.

Scanlon, P. W. *Split dose radiotherapy for bone and soft tissue sarcoma*, Am. J. Roent., 1972, **114**, 544.

Windeyer, B., Dische, S., and Mansfield, C. M. *The place of radiotherapy in the management of fibrosarcoma of the soft tissues*, 1966, **17**, 32.

15

Lympho-reticular System

The lymphomas appear to be malignant degeneration of different derivatives of a common stem cell. The four main varieties are Hodgkin's disease, lymphosarcoma, reticulum cell sarcoma and follicular lymphoma. They are closely related histologically and may be variants of the same disease, possibly with an immunological basis. The lymphomas represent about 5 per cent of all cancer.

In recent years a histological classification of the non-Hodgkin's lymphomas was described by Rappaport *et al.* (Table XI). This has several

TABLE XI

Non-Hodgkin's lymphomas (Rappaport)

Nodular (44%)	Diffuse (56%)
Histiocytic	Histiocytic
Mixed	Mixed
Lymphocytic, poorly differentiated	Lymphocytic, poorly differentiated
Lymphocytic, well differentiated	Lymphocytic, well differentiated
	Undifferentiated

advantages over the above orthodox classification. However it has not yet been fully accepted and indeed may be revised. For this reason the conventional classification is used in this discussion. It is noted however that most cases of giant follicular lymphoma fall into Rappaport's nodular group, whereas most cases of reticulum cell sarcoma are classified as diffuse histiocytic lymphomas.

HODGKIN'S DISEASE

This disease may occur at any age but is relatively more common in young people. The cause is unknown although many aetiological factors such as viruses have been suggested. Hodgkin's disease usually arises in a lymph gland in the neck and eventually spreads to involve lymph tissue throughout the body. The undoubted lasting cures obtained with Stage I lesions suggest that the disease is unifocal in origin (see also page 189).

Histology

The lymph node architecture is destroyed and replaced with sheets of pleomorphic cells. These include lymphocytes, reticulum cells, eosinophils and Reed-Sternberg cells. The Reed-Sternberg cell is usually considered pathognomonic of Hodgkin's disease although it has now been reported in other conditions. It is a giant cell with a pleomorphic cytoplasm and a large nucleus containing two or more nuclei. This bi-lobed nucleus is sometimes likened to an 'owl's eye'. It is often mitotic and is regarded by some as a reticulum cell; others consider it to be an abnormal histiocyte. Some pathologists have even suggested that it is a dead-end cell that does not proliferate. Histologists disagree about the classification of Hodgkin's disease. The old divisions of paragranuloma, granuloma and sarcoma are no longer recognized. Various alternative classifications have been devised to fit the microscopic appearance.

Luke's classification is widely used:

1 Lymphocytic — histiocytic. Five per cent.
2 Nodular sclerosis. Fifty per cent.
3 Mixed cell type. Forty per cent.
4 Lymphocytic depletion or Hodgkin's sarcoma. Five per cent.

Clinical Features

Most cases present with cervical lymph node enlargement. Axillary and inguinal nodes are affected initially in only 10 per cent of cases. The glands are usually painless, 'rubbery' and discrete. Patients usually have no other symptoms in the early stages.

Eventually involvement of the hilar, para-aortic and other glands may cause chest, abdominal and systemic symptoms. The clinical picture is subject to infinite variation owing to the widespread distribution of the lymphatic system.

There may also be an associated intermittent fever (Pel-Ebstein). Night sweating and lethargy are common complaints. Alcohol pain is a rare but well-recognized symptom in Hodgkin's disease.

On physical examination the patient may be in good general condition, but in the later stages he may be wasted and anaemic. The spleen and liver may be enlarged.

Stage

A simple classification into early localized and late generalized disease has been replaced by the following four stages:

I   Localized to one lymph node group.
II   Two neighbouring node groups involved.
III Lymph node involvement above and below diaphragm. The spleen is considered to be a lymph node.
IV   Generalized disease with organ involvement.

Each stage can be sub-divided into (*a*) patients with no systemic symptoms; (*b*) patients with systemic symptoms.

Investigations

1 Lymph node biopsy.
2 Chest X-ray.
3 Lymphangiogram.
4 Inferior vena cavogram and/or pyelogram.
5 Blood count.
6 Bone marrow biopsy.

Laparotomy and Splenectomy

The pre-operative assessment of disease below the diaphragm is often wrong. For this reason, many clinicians recommend laparotomy and splenectomy in young patients with Hodgkin's disease. However, these procedures are associated with some morbidity and, very rarely, mortality. Moreover, since laparotomy can delay the onset of potentially curative treatment by several weeks, it has been suggested that surgical exploration be postponed until the primary neck treatment has been completed.

Laparotomy is, of course, only indicated if the operative findings will influence the subsequent management of the patient.

Treatment

Radiotherapy is the treatment of choice for early disease. If the disease is confined to one lymph node group it may be completely cured.

Supervoltage therapy is recommended. Several techniques have been described:

LOCAL TREATMENT. This was used for many years. A simple 'trunk bridge' arrangement of four radiation fields to the neck was described. It was recommended that fields should cover at least 5 cm on either side of the palpable nodes. Many patients were cured using this method. A 'chasing' technique was then employed, using modest doses of radiation to local node groups if and when they appeared.

Local treatment is still indicated in frail elderly patients who are less able to tolerate extended field therapy.

MANTLE THERAPY. Larger fields to include all the nodes above the diaphragm are now being used in many centres (Figure 20). This so-called 'mantle' field covers both sides of the neck, both supraclavicular fossa, both axilla and the mediastinum. There are a number of problems in mantle dosimetry related to the geometry of the patient contour. Compensating filters are needed to ensure homogeneous irradiation. Care must be taken to include all lymph node drainage areas, especially the subclavian nodes, the pre-auricular nodes and the lower part of the axilla. Inadequate field coverage can result in marginal recurrence.

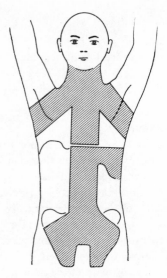

Figure 20   The mantle and inverted Y

INVERTED Y THERAPY. Radiation fields can be extended to cover all involved nodes below the diaphragm. These may include the para-aortic nodes and the iliac and inguinal areas. The splenic pedicle is sometimes included in this arrangement. In the young female it is difficult to protect ovarian tissue, and occasionally transposition of the ovaries has been recommended.

DOSE. Most cases of Hodgkin's disease are controlled locally with doses above 2500 rads in 2 to 3 weeks. It has been stated that the local recurrence rate is less than 1 per cent following a dose of 4500 rads in 4 to 5 weeks. But it is a law of diminishing returns, and there is probably little advantage in exceeding 3500 rads in 4 weeks. Published data on dosimetry should be scrutinized carefully. Analysis of fractionation and other factors may reveal considerable dosimetry differences between centres.

The prescribed doses in most instances are close to the limits of tolerance of the spinal cord, the tolerance of which is a function not only of dose but also of total length of cord irradiated. Other structures which should be protected during treatment include the laryngeal cartilages and the kidneys.

Currently the possibility of returning to smaller fields and lower doses in selected patients is being re-explored.

CHEMOTHERAPY. Cytotoxic drugs should never be used as the first line of attack in early Hodgkin's disease. Advanced disease, however, may be treated by a combination of radiotherapy and chemotherapy. Local swellings may shrink following small doses of palliative radiation. Chemotherapy may then control systemic symptoms for long periods of time. Nitrogen mustard, vincristine, procarbazine and prednisone (MOPP) are the most useful agents. There is evidence that better results are obtained with combination multiple drug therapy rather than sequential therapy with single drugs. This subject is discussed further in Chapter 24.

Treatment Policy
Various treatment policies are being tested. The following plan has been adopted in many centres.

Stage I   Mantle therapy: 4000 rads to involved nodes with 3000 rads to contiguous areas.

Stage II   Mantle therapy: 4000 rads to involved nodes with 3000 rads to contiguous areas. The upper para-aortic region is considered contiguous to the mediastinum.

Stage III   Mantle therapy followed by inverted Y therapy; similar dose levels are recommended but because of the large volumes of tissue involved, treatment must be fractionated over an extended period of time.

Stage IV   Chemotherapy. Local radiotherapy as required.

Results
Since pathologists disagree about the diagnosis of Hodgkin's disease in up to 20 per cent of cases, results of treatment should be interpreted with caution. The following 5-year survival rates are quoted:

Overall   = 40 per cent.
Stage I   = 80 per cent.
Stage II = 60 per cent.
Stage III = 40 per cent.
Stage IV = 15 per cent.

After 11 years the survival curve follows that of the general population. The prognosis is slightly better for young females with nodular sclerosis and for the lymphocytic predominant type of disease. Fever is a bad prognostic sign.

Complications
With conventional treatment, side-effects are transient and minimal. However, the more recent aggressive forms of therapy will inevitably produce some unwanted sequelae. Indiscriminate radiation therapy can produce serious damage including pericarditis, transverse myelitis, intestinal adhesions and leukaemia.

RETICULUM CELL SARCOMA

This disease usually occurs in patients over 60 years. Many features are similar to Hodgkin's disease, but glandular enlargement can be rapid and painful. There is often early involvement of the liver and bone marrow. Unlike Hodgkin's disease, reticulum cell sarcoma can present in other sites such as the tonsil, nasopharynx, bone or testes.

The normal lymph node architecture is obliterated. Histologically there is a bizarre pleomorphic picture with large pale mitotic reticulum cells. The tumour may resemble anaplastic carcinoma or merge with Hodgkin's disease.

For the purpose of treatment, it is convenient to use the same staging system as Hodgkin's disease. Many therapists also follow the same treatment policy with radiation to the primary lesion and lymph node drainage areas. This disease is slightly more radioresistant, and doses of up to 4500 rads in 4 to 5 weeks are required.

Primary lesions of bone are often localized and may sometimes be cured with radiation alone.

Results

Overall 5-year survival = 15 per cent.

Early disease = 60 per cent.

Further details are not yet available but it appears that an 8-year survival is compatible with complete cure. Stage for stage, the disease has a similar prognosis to Hodgkin's disease, but unfortunately many more patients present with advanced disease.

LYMPHOSARCOMA

This disease is slightly more common than reticulum cell sarcoma. Histologically, there is a mixed picture with lymphocytes interspersed between lymphoblasts. Either cell may predominate, but the lymphoblastic type carries the worst prognosis.

Again, lymphosarcoma has many of the features of Hodgkin's disease but lymphosarcoma may also present in the nasopharynx, orbit, neck, mediastinum, stomach or intestine. The treatment of choice is also radiotherapy, and a Hodgkin's type policy may be followed. Doses of up to 3500 rads in 3 to 4 weeks are usually sufficient to prevent local recurrence. Unlike Hodgkin's disease, the natural history of lymphosarcoma suggests a multifocal or systemic disease.

Results

Overall 5-year survival = 20 per cent.

Early disease = 65 per cent.

After 8 years the survival curve again follows that of the general population.

Most patients present with advanced disease, but occasional prolonged remissions have been reported without any form of treatment. Combinations of whole body radiation and chemotherapy are presently under investigation.

Stage for stage, the survival rates for Hodgkin's disease and lymphosarcoma are similar although again Hodgkin's disease has a better overall prognosis because more cases present at an earlier stage.

FOLLICULAR LYMPHOMA

Giant cell follicular lymphoma or Brill-Symmer's disease is the least aggressive malignant disease of the lympho-reticular system. Nevertheless it requires early treatment for complete eradication. The clinical features are similar to those of Hodgkin's disease, and the condition may be classified in the same way. The tumour is highly radiosensitive, and doses of up to 3000 rads in 3 weeks are often sufficient to control local disease. The overall 5-year survival is 65 per cent but about one half of all cases will eventually develop a more malignant form of lymphoma, usually lymphosarcoma. A number of cases of spontaneous regression have been noted. Women have a better prognosis than men.

PRE-MALIGNANT LYMPHOMA

The histological diagnosis of lymphoma is often equivocal. In many of these patients the clinical picture is identical to Hodgkin's disease. A series of almost 500 cases has been collected in Manchester. These patients were treated by radiotherapy even though the microscopic diagnosis of lymphoma had not been confirmed. The interesting fact emerged that stage for stage, the survival was the same as for Hodgkin's disease.

BURKITT'S LYMPHOMA

This tumour of African children has been reported in other countries. Some histologists believe it is a form of lymphosarcoma. The disease is unknown in the first year of life and is uncommon in adults. However, it has been reported in adults and Europeans entering endemic areas for the first time. The disease is associated with the Ebstein-Barr virus which causes infectious mononucleosis elsewhere. The reason for this is obscure but it may be related to immunological defence mechanisms.

In over half the cases, the primary tumour involves the jaw, but the disease is often widespread. The most advanced stages involve the nervous system. Burkitt's lymphoma is highly radiosensitive. Unfortunately, radiotherapy is not available in many parts of Africa, and its role in this disease has not been fully explored. There is evidence however that early disease responds to small doses of radiation therapy to the localized tumour mass,

Chemotherapy is used extensively and is curative in many cases. Cytoxan therapy is the drug of choice. Various dose schedules are being tested, and the reader is referred to the latest literature for up-to-date recommendations.

It is difficult to give an exact prognosis since long-term follow-up is impossible in Africa and, in any case, an estimated 20 per cent of children in Uganda die before the age of 3 from other causes. However, long-term recovery following chemotherapy, together with spontaneous regressions have been well documented. Recent reports suggest that the overall survival rate is over 30 per cent.

HISTIOCYTOSIS X

Eosinophilic granuloma, Hand-Schuller-Christian disease and Letterer-Siwe disease have been classified as a single nosological entity, histiocytosis X. There is some evidence that these conditions should not be grouped together, but the classification is used here for convenience until a better one is found.

The disease is mainly found in children.

Histology

The histiocyte is a mobile phagocytic cell found in the tissues. This 'wandering histiocyte' has the ability to become a mononuclear macrophage in an emergency. Histiocytosis X is a malignant proliferation of these cells.

The lesion consists of a histiocytic granuloma containing a pathological histiocyte with a large distorted nucleus and granules in the cytoplasm. Around the granuloma there is an intense reaction with an eosinophilic infiltrate.

Classification

TYPE I: CHRONIC LOCALIZED TYPE. Patients usually present with bone pain. Radiographs show early bone lesions with areas of rarefaction. This disease was formerly called eosinophilic granuloma of bone.

TYPE II: CHRONIC GENERALIZED TYPE. More advanced lesions usually involve lungs. Patients may present with dyspnoea or pneumothorax. Examination often reveals finger clubbing with diffuse, bilateral, symmetrical millet-seed reticulation in the middle and upper lung fields. This often proceeds to honeycombing. Patients have a raised sedimentation rate. Lesions may also involve other viscera, and there may be punched-out bony defects in the skull. These may produce the triad of exophthalmos, diabetes insipidus and cranial abnormalities. This syndrome has been labelled Hand-Schuller-Christian disease.

TYPE III: ACUTE DISSEMINATED TYPE. Advanced malignant phase. This is usually found in infants and young children. Widespread multiple involvement including the skin carries the eponym Letterer-Siwe disease.

Diagnosis

Biopsy must be obtained since there are a number of other diseases that produce cystic bone lesions.

Treatment

Radiotherapy is recommended for localized disease with bone destruction. Small doses up to 1000 rads in six treatments are usually sufficient to prevent local recurrence. Radiation is also valuable for palliation of distressing skin lesions in young children. Generalized disease calls for a systemic approach with steroids and cytotoxic agents.

Results

Type I	5-year survival = 80 per cent.
Type II	5-year survival = 40 per cent.
Type III	5-year survival = less than 5 per cent.

MAST CELL DISEASE

Mast cells are involved in the metabolism of serotonin, histamine and heparin. Mast cell disease is grouped with the lymphomas for convenience.

1 Urticara Pigmentosa

This skin disorder begins in childhood but regresses in puberty. Mast cells are found in the epidermis. Patients complain of episodes of red flushing and fainting. The disease is benign, although there is a rare lethal cutaneous variety which causes necrosis of small blood vessels. The results of radiotherapy are under investigation.

2 Systemic Mastocytosis

This rare disease occurs in adults. It resembles the other lymphomas but often presents with bleeding episodes due to an abnormality in heparin metabolism. Other clinical features may include malabsorption and bone changes. Symptomatic treatment with blood transfusion, antihistamines and steroids is recommended. Occasionally radiation is of value.

LYMPHOMAS OF SKIN (see Chapter 6)

References

Easson, E. *Modern Trends in Radiotherapy*, ed. Deely and Wood, 1967, **1**, 277.
Kaplan, H. *Hodgkin's disease*, Harvard University Press, Boston, 1972.
Rappaport, H., Winter, W. J., and Hicks, E. B. Follicular lymphoma. In *Management of Hodgkin's Disease and the Other Lymphomas*, ed. E. S. Greenwald and W. Zeitlin, Medical Examination Publishing Company, Inc., New York, 1971, pp 23-52.
The Hodgkin Maze, The Lancet, 4 October 1969 and 22 May 1971.

16

Blood Disorders

The role of radiation therapy in the management of malignant blood diseases varies from year to year. As a background to these changes, some current concepts on general management are discussed below.

Polycythaemia

Polycythaemia may be defined as an abnormal increase in the number of circulating red cells or an increase in the total red cell mass. This may be primary or secondary. Secondary polycythaemia is due to an increased level of erythropoietin. This may be an appropriate response to a physiological stimulus such as hypoxia in chronic pulmonary disease.

In secondary polycythaemia there is usually no splenomegaly, thrombocytosis or leukocytosis. The treatment is that of the primary disorder.

Polycythaemia Vera

This disease is one of the myeloproliferative disorders, the others being chronic myeloid leukaemia, thrombocythaemia, Di Guglielmo's syndrome and myelosclerosis. In primary polycythaemia, an inappropriate increase in erythropoiesis is present due to the autonomous production of red cells by the marrow without increased erythropoietin production. There is an associated proliferation of leucoblastic and megakaryocytic tissue. The red cell count, white cell count and platelet count are all usually increased. Haemoglobin, packed cell volume and leukocyte alkaline phosphatase are all raised. Blood viscosity is increased, and red cell life may be shortened.

CLINICAL FEATURES. The onset of the disease is insidious. Patients are usually elderly and have a characteristic rubicund appearance with a dusky cyanosis.

A variety of symptoms and signs are found due to the abnormal blood picture. Most patients complain of intense itching following a hot bath. Ischaemic episodes involving the heart, brain or limbs may occur. Splenomegaly is a common finding.

Paradoxically, polycythaemic patients can present with anaemia. This may be due to haemorrhage from a peptic ulcer or to bone marrow exhaustion. Secondary gout is sometimes seen.

TREATMENT. 1. Repeated venesection is the first line of treatment for all patients. Patients can become iron deficient, however. This may not be apparent unless the MCV is measured at regular intervals.

2. If frequent venesection is required to control the disease, it is usually necessary to give some form of marrow depressant. There is little to choose between radioactive phosphorus (P^{32}) and cytotoxic drugs. The survival following each form of treatment is about the same, although the mode of death may be different. It has been argued that P^{32} is a more convenient form of therapy since the patient is not required to take a lengthy course of tablets. The dose of P^{32} is usually about four millicuries. It can be given orally or intravenously. If the oral route is used, the dose should be somewhat higher to allow for lower absorption from the intestinal tract.

Alkylating agents may also be used. Chlorambucil (6 to 8 mg daily) or Cyclophosphamide (100 to 150 mg daily) have both been recommended. Diminution in white cell and platelet count are the first effects observed. The response in haematocrit follows in about three to four months. Once the haematocrit has been stabilized at normal levels, maintenance therapy using approximately one half of the induction dose is instituted.

3. Whole body irradiation was formerly given to these patients but the technique has now been virtually abandoned in favour of the above methods of treatment.

RESULTS. The average life expectation is about 13 years. This is almost equal to the normal life expectancy for patients in the age groups affected. Twenty per cent of cases terminate in a leukaemic phase. The remainder die from other causes.

CHRONIC MYELOID LEUKAEMIA

Most patients with chronic myeloid or granulocytic leukaemia present in middle age with an insidious onset of symptoms, a progressively enlarging spleen and anaemia. The disease differs from the other myeloproliferative disorders in that it is associated with a defect in the long arm of autosome 22. This genetic hallmark is known as the Philadelphia chromosome and is found in 90 per cent of patients. It is an abnormality of the myeloid stem cell and is also found in other marrow elements including the red cells and platelets.

The blood picture usually shows a 'shift to the left' with immature blast cells and a corresponding marrow picture. The white cell count may be raised above 200 000. The platelet count is raised at first but later there may be thrombocytopenia due to marrow hypoplasia. At this stage there may be an attempt at extramedullary haemopoesis. A striking biochemical abnormality is the reduction in leukocyte alkaline phosphatase. Associated with this, marked elevations of serum vitamin B-12 are sometimes seen.

Treatment

Initially most patients respond to cytotoxic drugs. The aim is to control the total granulocytic mass. This is considered to be out of control when there is gross hepatosplenomegaly or a high white cell count.

Many drugs are effective in the early stages of the disease. Currently busulphan is a drug of choice. A dose of 4 mg daily has been recommended. Care should be taken not to suppress the marrow completely. To ensure this, the fall in white cell count can be plotted on semi-logarithmic graph paper and the optimum drug dose predicted. A reduction of white cell count to about 10 000 is considered satisfactory, but often patients are stabilized at 20 000.

Blood transfusion may be required if the haemoglobin or platelets drop precipitously. Sometimes patients develop secondary gout requiring symptomatic treatment.

Radiotherapy is no longer considered to be the first line of attack in this disease although it may be used to control massive splenomegaly causing discomfort. Treatment should be given cautiously initially since some patients are unduly sensitive even to small doses of radiation. A starting dose of about 50 rads is recommended. This may be increased daily according to the patient's response. A total dose of 2000 rads is usually adequate to control symptoms.

Results

The average survival time is 3 to 4 years. This is really little better than the results of 50 years ago. Although the duration of survival is not impressive, patients usually obtain considerable symptomatic relief and feel well. The disease usually terminates in a short acute blastic cell crisis. At this stage, treatment is of little effect although many drugs are currently being studied.

The side-effects of busulphan are important in this disease and are discussed later (see Chapter 24).

CHRONIC LYMPHOCYTIC LEUKAEMIA

This disease usually presents in patients over 45 years. There are no generally accepted criteria for the diagnosis of this slowly progressive condition. Generalized adenopathy, splenomegaly, a peripheral blood count of more than 15 000 lymphocytes/mm³ and a marrow containing 50 per cent lymphocytes are typical. In the florid case, the white cell count may be elevated to levels of 30 000 to 500 000 with 90 per cent lymphocytes. But there are many cases which lack the typical findings. Some haematologists would include patients with a low or normal white cell count but relative lymphocytosis as 'sub-leukaemic' cases.

Eventually the total mass of lymphocytes infiltrates the lymph nodes, bone marrow, spleen and liver causing suppression of platelets, neutrophils and red cells. The lymph node histology is indistinguishable from lymphocytic lymphosarcoma which may be a variant of the same disease. There is often an associated immunoparesis accompanied by hypersplenism and an auto-immune haemolytic anaemia.

There appears to be a continuous spectrum between typical chronic lymphocytic leukaemia with small compact cells, and lymphosarcoma-cell leukaemia with large cleaved nucleated cells.

Treatment

The difficulty in diagnosis of this disease is also reflected in disagreement about the indications for therapy. It has been suggested that some patients may require no treatment apart from occasional blood transfusion to control anaemia and general measures to combat infection. Others advocate treatment for all patients whether they have indolent or aggressive disease.

Chlorambucil is the drug of choice. A dose of 12 mg per day is effective if carefully monitored. It is recommended that this be given up to the point of mild haematopoietic toxicity and maintained for at least 12 weeks.

Cortisone is indicated if there is an associated auto-immune disorder. It suppresses lymphocyte production without repressing the bone marrow. It also has a lympholytic action. In marrow failure, a daily dose of 40 mg of Prednisone is recommended. This can be gradually reduced after 2 months if the marrow recovers.

Radiation therapy is indicated if lymph nodes are causing pressure symptoms. Where small volumes of tissue are being irradiated, a dose of 2000 rads in 2 weeks is usually adequate. Larger fields require more protracted therapy.

Massive splenomegaly causing abdominal discomfort may be treated with splenic irradiation. This can be given conveniently through anterior and posterior fields directed to the left upper quadrant. Again, treatment should be started cautiously with doses of about 50 rads per day. This may be increased gradually if the blood count permits. The dose and field size can be tailored to the response of the spleen and peripheral blood count. A final total dose of 2000 rads is usually sufficient.

Results

Overall 5-year survival = 50 per cent.

Most clinicians feel that treatment prolongs life, but this is difficult to prove since the disease is often relatively benign, especially in the elderly.

Growth-rate kinetic studies indicate that the lymphocytes in this disease are long-lived although the rate of lymphocyte production is approximately normal. Studies also suggest that there are probably two types of disease; one with a 5-year survival of 80 per cent, and the other with a 5-year survival of 40 per cent.

There is some evidence that a normal population of lymphocytes persists and that these cells are more resistant to drugs. If so, we may yet find better means of controlling the disease by exploiting this differential drug sensitivity.

ACUTE LEUKAEMIA

Acute myelogenous leukaemia is mainly a disease of adults. At the present time, radiation therapy plays no part in the management of this disease. However, survival has recently improved from 2 months to over 1 year, and it is possible that radiation may yet have a part to play.

Acute lymphoblastic leukaemia is a disease of childhood. Until recently this was considered a fatal disease. Happily a few long-term survivors are now being obtained with chemotherapy.

The place of radiation therapy has changed over the years. Formerly, whole body radiation was used, but as newer drugs were discovered, radiation therapy was used less and less. In recent years, however, there has been a revival of interest in irradiation. As patients survive longer, there is an increased incidence of meningeal leukaemia which may produce neck stiffness and distressing associated symptoms, including cranial nerve palsies. Small doses of palliative radiation often provide dramatic relief for these patients.

The blood-brain barrier is a pharmacological 'hideout', and for this reason it has now been proposed that patients in remission should be given a course of prophylactic irradiation to the entire neuraxis in an attempt to prolong life. Various dose schedules have been prescribed ranging from 1200 to 2400 rads in 2 to 3 weeks.

It has been suggested that a combined therapeutic attack on acute leukaemia could improve the long-term prognosis from 15 to 50 per cent. If this proves to be true, then radiation therapy should not be given as a palliative measure but rather with the meticulous care presently devoted to, for instance, a case of medulloblastoma.

HYPERSPLENISM

In this syndrome the spleen is enlarged and there is increased splenic destruction of red cells, white cells and platelets.

Fewer idiopathic cases are described as more causes are elucidated. These include lymphomas, Gaucher's disease and kala azar.

The treatment of choice is the treatment of the primary condition. If pancytopenia is severe, it may be necessary to resort to splenectomy. Where surgery is contra-indicated, radiation therapy is a useful alternative. Often the spleen is unduly sensitive to radiation, and small doses should be used starting with 25 rads daily, increasing gradually to a maximum total dose of 1000 rads (see also page 119).

MULTIPLE MYELOMA

This disease is included here for convenience. It is discussed in more detail for two reasons: firstly, radiotherapists see a lot of myeloma; secondly, many therapists are involved with the chemotherapeutic management of this condition.

Multiple myeloma is due to the malignant proliferation of plasma cells. The disease is grouped with the monoclonal immunopathies and is classified according to the type of immunoglobulin produced.

Chemical Pathology

Infections provoke a broad spectrum antibody response giving a wide band of gammaglobulin on paper electrophoresis. These antibodies can be sub-divided and separated immunologically into homogeneous proteins or M-Components, each containing a heavy molecular chain (G, A, M, D or E) and a light molecular chain (K or L).

A solitary narrow electrophoretic band is occasionally a healthy antibody response; more often it means that a monoclone of cells is reproducing itself in a neoplastic manner. These cells may be de-differentiated and produce an excess of heavy chains, light chains or chain fragments. Light chains are small and appear in the urine as Bence-Jones proteins (BJP).

A solitary M-Component may be normal in 25 per cent of patients. The remainder of cases are due to:

1 Multiple myeloma. This accounts for 50 per cent of cases. The disease is classified as Ig G, Ig A, Ig M, Ig E, Ig D or Bence-Jones myelomatosis. Ig G and Ig A are the most common types. A few highly malignant clones are so anaplastic that they produce no paraprotein at all.

2 Malignant lymphomas.

3 Waldenstrom's macroglobulinaemia. This rare disease is mainly due to Ig M.

4 Heavy chain disease. This very rare condition is usually found in men.

By measuring the level of M-Component at different times, it is possible to study plasma cell kinetics and assess whether a clone is benign or malignant. It is also possible to measure the degree of malignancy and the response to treatment.

Histology

The tumour is composed of sheets of typical and atypical plasma cells called myeloma cells. They have a small dense eccentric nucleus with a spoke or clock-like chromatin pattern. The cells may be well differentiated, moderately differentiated or anaplastic. Eventually there is a diffuse cellular infiltration of the bone marrow.

Stage
The following staging system is a convenient method of classifying plasma cell malignancy:

    I   Plasmacytoma. This localized plasma cell tumour may be: (a) medullary; (b) extra-medullary (15 per cent of cases).
   II   Myeloma (most cases).
 III   Plasma cell leukaemia (very rare).

Clinical Features
Multiple myeloma occurs mainly in middle-aged and elderly people. Bone lesions are present in 80 per cent of cases. Pain is a common symptom, and pathological fractures are frequently found. Most patients are anaemic and develop associated infections due to immunoparesis. Hypercalcaemia is also relatively common. Many patients terminate in renal failure. Miscellaneous features include amyloidosis, peripheral neuritis and gout.

Investigations
  1 X-ray may show:
        a   Osteoporosis.
        b   Discrete 'punched-out' osteolytic lesions; 'Pepper pot' skull.
        c   Pathological fractures.
        d   Preservation of the vertebral pedicles.
        e   Involvement of the mandible.
  2 Bone marrow biopsy. Contains more than 20 per cent plasma cells.
  3 Sedimentation rate is very high.
  4 Blood picture.
  5 Electrophoresis.
  6 Immunoglobulins. The M-Component is greater than 2 g per cent.

Treatment
Plasmacytoma is a potentially curable tumour. The lesion is radiosensitive and responds to a dose of about 4000 rads in 3 weeks. The field size depends on the extent of the lesion, but an adequate margin should be allowed.

The management of multiple myeloma is a complex problem and involves general measures with the judicious use of radiation therapy for painful bony lesions. Patients may require blood transfusion for severe anaemia, dialysis for renal failure and antibiotics to combat infection.

The bone lesions are usually radiosensitive and respond to doses of radiation varying from 1250 rads in a single treatment to 2100 rads in three treatments. The fractionation depends on patient tolerance and the volume of tissue irradiated. If pain relief is not obtained inside 1 week, it often means that the symptoms are due to associated osteoporosis rather than myeloma. Pathological rib fractures create a difficult therapeutic problem because of the constant movement of the rib cage, but even these lesions respond to small doses of radiation. Care should be taken to avoid irradiation of underlying lung tissue, and electron therapy is often helpful for this purpose.

Combination drug therapy is superior to single agents. 'Pulsed' chemotherapy has been studied in an attempt to attack the disease during the most sensitive part of the cell cycle. Melphalan, vincristine, prednisone and procarbazine have all been used (see also Chapter 24).

Results

The 5-year survival for localized plasmacytoma is 60 per cent.

Ten years ago the average life expectancy for multiple myeloma was 18 months and the 2-year survival 20 per cent. Since then the prognosis has improved considerably and the 2-year survival is now over 70 per cent. It appears that this improved survival depends more on careful follow-up of patients and judicious therapeutic intervention, rather than on the discovery of new drugs.

The Ig type of disease has no influence on prognosis but a poor outlook is associated with the following: serum albumin of less than 4 g per cent; blood urea greater than 80 mg per cent; Bence-Jones protein greater than 200 mg per cent; a haemoglobin less than 7·5 g; poorly differentiated lesions.

The palliative value of radiation therapy is considerable and most patients obtain dramatic relief of pain following treatment.

SPLENOMEGALY

The spleen may be enlarged in the lymphoproliferative disorders due to hypersplenism, tumour invasion or extramedullary haematopoiesis. In the latter event, the spleen is doing a normal job and splenic irradiation may be dangerous. Thus it is important to start with a low dose and proceed cautiously as already indicated.

Myelofibrosis and myeolidmetaplasia (MMM) is a slowly progressive syndrome characterized by overgrowth of haemotopoietic and connective tissue in the marrow and reticuloendothelial system. It is a complex disease and has over 20 synonyms. Cautious radiotherapy to the spleen may sometimes be indicated in the management of this disease.

References

Gilbert, H., and Dameshek, W. *The myeloproliferative disorders*, Disease-a-Month, October 1970.
Spiers, A. S. D. *Acute Leukaemia*, The Lancet, 1972, **2**, 473.

17

Female Genital Tract

CARCINOMA OF THE CERVIX

Aetiology

Cancer of the cervix is more common in multiparous women, possibly due to trauma and chronic cervicitis. Early promiscuity may be a factor in some cases; the disease is common in prostitutes and unknown in nuns. Coital hygiene may also play a part; the disease is rare in Jewesses and has been related to male circumcision. The condition is relatively common in lower-income groups. An association is suspected with herpes virus Type 2. Cancer of the cervix occurs mainly in the age group of 45 to 55, but it is also found in younger women. It is particularly common in underdeveloped countries.

Pathology

Most tumours are squamous carcinomas arising from the squamous-columnar junction. About 5 per cent are adenocarcinomas from the endocervix, but they behave in the same way as squamous lesions.

The tumour spreads by direct extension to the vaginal fornices and laterally to the broad ligament. Here it may erode a large blood vessel or obstruct the lower end of a ureter. It may also spread to the vagina or to the body of the uterus. Anterior and posterior spread is less common.

Lymphatic spread may involve the obturator, iliac, sacral, peri-aortic and even supraclavicular nodes. Retrograde spread to the inguinal nodes may occur. Blood spread is late.

There is evidence that invasive carcinoma of the cervix develops from a field of atypical epithelium and not from a single cell. The peak incidence of carcinoma-in-situ occurs at 35 years and that of invasive carcinoma at 45.

Stage

The following stages are recognized:

- o Pre-invasive, intra-epithelial carcinoma-in-situ.
- I Confined to cervix.
- II Extension to upper third of vagina or broad ligament.

III Extension to lower third of vagina or lateral pelvic wall. (On rectal examination no 'cancer-free' space is palpable between tumour and pelvic wall).

IV Involving bladder, rectum or distant metastases.

Clinical Features

The patient usually presents with a blood-stained vaginal discharge which may be post-coital. Frank bleeding may lead to anaemia. Pyometra may occur. Urinary symptoms vary from mild frequency to uraemia. Pelvic pain is usually a late symptom. Advanced disease may present with fistula formation or metastases.

Investigations

The diagnosis can usually be made by pelvic examination, but a biopsy should always be obtained. This should be combined with curettage and excision of the endocervix. Schiller's test can be used for early cases. This consists of painting the cervix with Schiller's iodine solution; normal tissue glycogen stains brown. Biopsy should be taken from the pale areas.

Blood count, blood urea and chest X-ray are essential. Complete assessment calls for cystoscopy, proctoscopy and intravenous pyelography. Lymphangiography may sometimes be helpful.

Exfoliative Cytology

Epithelial cells desquamated from the genital tract may be collected from the posterior fornix of the vagina with a bulb pipette. Cervical smears may be taken with Ayre's spatula and stained with Papinicolaou's stain. Malignancy is suggested by bizarre pleomorphic small cells, increased nuclear-cytoplasmic ratio, a thick irregular nuclear membrane and mitotic figures. The test is never diagnostic, and a positive smear demands full investigation. Even if curettage and biopsy are negative, one must realize that a neoplasm may be concealed in a fallopian tube. False negative results are also obtained, thus women with symptoms must always be referred to a gynaecologist for fuller investigation. It is important to appreciate that the cervical smear is only a mass screening test for symptomless women. A single test in a patient's lifetime is of little value. Smears should be repeated at least every 3 years. Although the detection rate is low, the test is economically worthwhile if it is reserved for those patients at special risk.

Treatment

General therapeutic measures are very important in this disease, and one should attempt to correct anaemia and control infection before embarking on treatment.

Cancer of the cervix is one of the most important diseases in radiotherapeutic practice, and the definitive role of radiation will be discussed first.

E

RADIOTHERAPY. This is the first line of attack in most cases of invasive carcinoma. Two essentially different techniques have been used, both employing radium and external radiation. The conventional system, which originated mainly in Manchester, will be described first.

(1) *Conventional Technique.* Early disease is often treated with a radium insertion alone. More advanced disease is treated with a combination of radium and external irradiation.

A thin tube of radium is inserted into the cervical canal after dilation under anaesthesia. A self-retaining catheter may be inserted to obviate the necessity for catheterization later on the ward. Two 'ovoids' of radium are carefully packed below the uterine tube in the right and left lateral fornices.

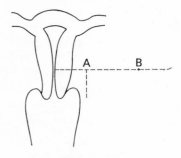

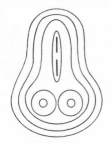

Figure 21
Point A and Point B

Figure 22
Isodose distribution

The 'ovoids' are separated by a washer or 'spacer'. The insertion is carried out in the knee-elbow position. This exposes the vaginal part of the tumour, facilitates dilation of the cervical canal and tends to antevert the mobile uterus. It also allows the radium to be loaded away from the rectum. A probe counter may be used to record the bladder and rectal dose. Finally the position of the radium is checked by X-ray examination.

No useful radium dosage can be prescribed at the external os or at the mucosa of the vaginal vault. In these regions the radiation intensity is high but falls off rapidly over distances of a few millimeters. The anatomical site chosen for prescription purposes is the paracervical triangle at the medial edge of the broad ligament where the uterine vessels cross the ureter. This is defined as an arbitrary geometrical point 2 cm lateral to the uterine canal and 2 cm up from the mucous membrane of the lateral fornix. It is called Point A. The dose of Point A is about equal to the dose at the rectovaginal septum and is the limiting dose. An additional point, Point B, has been defined 3 cm lateral to Point A. Point B approximates to the obturator node (Figure 21).

The isodose lines are designed to follow the spread of the disease, and are shaped like a 'flat pear' (Figure 22).

The recommended dose is 8000 rads to Point A and 3500 rads to Point B. (The uterine wall probably receives about 30 000 rads and the vaginal wall 25 000 rads.) There are various ways of achieving this (Manchester, Stockholm and Paris techniques) depending on the total time and fractionation of the insertions. A suitable method is two separate 70-hour insertions of radium, 1 week apart.

The radium loading of the tubes and ovoids is as shown in (Figure 23). The object is to insert the longest tube and the largest ovoids that will fit snugly in position. This ensures that the dose fall-off is not too rapid. The loading is designed to give the same dose at Point A, regardless of the length of the applicator. However, small ovoids lower the dose at Point B by about 10 per cent, and a short tube lowers the dose at Point A. Furthermore, if the ovoids are inserted in tandem the dose at Point A is lowered by 8 per cent.

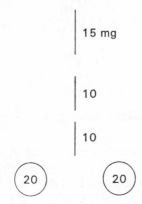

Figure 23   Radium loading: conventional technique

Stage III and IV lesions require supplementary external megavoltage radiation. This is usually directed to the parametria through 2 pairs of parallel opposed fields measuring about 12 × 5 cm. An additional 3000 rads in three weeks is prescribed to the midline overlying Point B. In these cases the total radium contribution to Point A should be reduced to 6500 rads.

Occasionally the external os is obscured by tumour when the patient is first seen. In such an event, vaginal radium only is inserted. Usually the os can be identified with ease 2 weeks later. Preliminary vaginal radium may also be indicated in an attempt to control haemorrhage or where perforation has occurred.

In the presence of gross pyometria, it may be necessary to delay treatment until drainage and antibiotic therapy have been instituted. In frail elderly patients the overall dose should be reduced by about 10 per cent.

Afterloading techniques are discussed later.

(2) *American Technique*. In recent years, the above plan has been modified in many centres, mainly in the USA. The modified technique involves greater reliance on external radiation to the total pelvis and personalization of each case. The dose is thus tailored to the individual patient. For instance, extension to the left parametrium calls for a greater dose to that side. Moreover, intracavitary radium employing a fixed geometry is replaced by versatile radium applicators allowing appropriate dosimetry. Occasionally an interstitial radium implant is used.

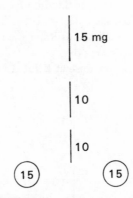

Figure 24   Radium loading: American technique

Early Stage I tumours may be treated by radium alone to a maximum dose of 10 000 mg hours. More advanced tumours are usually treated by whole pelvis radiation in the first instance. This tends to contract the tumour tissue volume towards the midline, making the subsequent radium insertion more effective. At the same time it avoids the problem of matching parametrial fields with a radium insertion which may be off-centre. The dose is usually taken to 4000 rads in 4 weeks through anterior and posterior portals measuring about 15 × 15 cm. Additional radiation up to 1500 rads may be given to the parametrium if required. This may be followed by a radium insertion of 5500 mg hours distributed as shown in Figure 24. Accurate dosimetry is essential since these dose levels are close to the limits of tolerance. It is recommended that at no time should the dose to the total pelvis exceed 5000 rads in 5 weeks. If higher doses are required, the field sizes should be reduced.

The Fletcher-Bloedorn applicators used in this system are cumbersome and protrude between the patient's legs. However, they allow adjustments to be made in the spatial dosimetry later if necessary. Moreover, they also permit the use of afterloading techniques using radium or caesium.

Surgery
The treatment of choice for carcinoma-in-situ is simple vaginal or abdominal hysterectomy. Cone biopsy may be recommended for young nulliparous

women with Stage o lesions who still wish to have children. It is essential, however, to obtain histological confirmation that the disease has been removed completely. Rarely, an intravaginal application of superficial X-ray therapy is required. This is indicated if Schiller's test suggests that the area of abnormal epithelium would otherwise demand cervical amputation, rather than cone resection. This technique calls for careful follow-up and hysterectomy when the patient's family is complete.

Wertheim's radical abdominal hysterectomy consists of removal of the uterus, tubes, ovaries, broad ligaments and parametrium, the upper two-thirds of the vagina and the regional lymph nodes. This procedure is occasion-ally indicated for Stage I and II lesions, although in most instances radio-therapy gives equally good if not better results, with lower morbidity and negligible mortality.

Absolute indications for radical surgery include poor response to radia-tion, extension to the corpus, uncontrollable sepsis, fistula, and anatomical abnormalities such as fibroids, which preclude proper radium insertion. Adenocarcinoma of the cervix is not an indication for surgery.

In advanced disease a defunctioning colostomy is sometimes necessary to relieve distressing symptoms. Intractable pain occasionally necessitates chordotomy. Anterior, posterior or total exenteration of the pelvis is a heroic procedure with a high mortality. It is sometimes justified in carefully selected patients. Primary tumours that invade in an anterior and posterior direction with little lateral spread are best suited for these ultra-radical procedures.

Results

Overall 5-year survival = 45 per cent.
Stage o   = 100 per cent.
Stage I   = 75 per cent.
Stage II   = 50 per cent.
Stage III   = 30 per cent.
Stage IV   = 5 per cent.

Somewhat better results are quoted for the 'personalized' American techniques. After 6 years, the survival curve follows that of the general population. Patients surviving without evident disease beyond this time can be considered cured. Recent work has shown that prognosis is worse if there is an abnormal chromosome number in the malignant cells. On the other hand, prognosis is improved if there are mast cells in the surrounding tissues.

Even where cure is not achieved, advanced bleeding lesions can often be controlled for many years with palliative radiation.

Complications

Early radiation effects on the bowel and bladder usually subside following symptomatic treatment. Late complications after high dose irradiation include rectal ulceration and fistula formation. Damage to the neck of the femur may lead to pathological fracture, but this can be prevented using diamond-shaped radiation fields avoiding the femur.

Stump Carcinoma

By definition a true stump carcinoma occurs 2 years or more after a supra-vaginal hysterectomy, the lesion having developed since surgery. A coincident stump carcinoma is due to residual tumour and occurs in under 2 years. These tumours lie close to the bladder and rectum. Because there is no uterine canal for intracavitary radium, stump carcinoma is best treated by external irradiation, followed by interstitial radium or transvaginal ortho-voltage radiotherapy. Survival rates of 50 per cent are quoted.

CARCINOMA OF THE ENDOMETRIUM

Aetiology

This tumour occurs mostly in women between 50 and 60 years. It often arises after a late menopause. Fifty per cent of the patients are nulliparous or infertile. The disease is associated with fibroids, diabetes mellitus and the oestrogen-secreting thecoma of the ovary.

Pathology

The lesion is usually an adenocarcinoma which may be well differentiated or anaplastic. An increasing number of squamous carcinomas and adeno-acanthomas have been reported.

Rare cases of sarcoma have also been described. These may occur following radiation-induced menopause or years after successful radium treatment for carcinoma of the cervix. Another rare variety is sarcoma botryoides (see soft tissue tumours, Chapter 14).

The line of spread depends partly on whether the tumour is in the upper or lower half of the uterus. The former extends directly through the muscle coat. The latter spreads to the cervix, vagina or ovaries. The lymph channels run to the iliac nodes, the round ligament, the inguinal glands, ovaries and the peri-aortic nodes. Blood spread is late.

Staging

The conventional international staging system has been unsatisfactory, and the following classification has been recommended:

   I   Corpus only.
   II   Enlarged uterus, greater than 7 cm.
   III Cervix involved.
   IV   Pelvic spread. Metastases.

One stage to be added for undifferentiated anaplastic lesions.

Clinical Features

Post-menopausal bleeding must be assumed to be due to cancer of the uterus until proved otherwise. In menopausal women, irregular bleeding may be the presenting symptom.

Investigations

    Blood picture.
    Chest X-ray and intravenous pyelogram.
    Fractional curettage and biopsy.
    Hysterography.
    Cystoscopy.
    Sigmoidoscopy.

Treatment

1. SURGERY. Total abdominal hysterectomy and bilateral salpingo-oophorectomy is the treatment of choice. This may be combined with radiotherapy.

2. RADIOTHERAPY. Most patients present with Stage I disease. In these cases, radiotherapy improves the overall survival by about 15 per cent, mainly by preventing vault recurrence. There is little to choose between pre-operative and post-operative radium in these cases. Details are given below.

At higher stages, radiotherapy markedly improves survival. Pre-operative radiation is preferred. It reduces the bulk of the growth and allows time to prepare the patient for hysterectomy. Two techniques have been described.

In the Manchester system, the technique is similar to that used in carcinoma of the cervix except that the ovoid loading is reduced and the uterine tube is thicker, measuring 1 cm in diameter. In cervical cancer the object is to throw the dose laterally, but in corpus tumours the object is to irradiate the uterine wall and upper third of the vagina. Thus the intra-uterine tubes carry between 40 and 65 mg of radium and the ovoids between 15 and 25 mg. The uterine sound is used to estimate the size of the uterine cavity beforehand for the appropriate-sized applicator; it is usually larger than in carcinoma of the cervix. The vaginal ovoids are generally inserted in tandem, but if there is cervical invasion they are placed in the lateral fornices. If surgery is contra-indicated for any reason, a full radical dose of 8000 rads to point A is given. This can be given conveniently in two 72-hour radium insertions, 1 week apart. If surgery is contemplated, however, the dose is reduced to two-thirds of a radical dose. In more advanced lesions, external radiation may be added to both parametrial areas.

In the USA, many therapists prefer to use Heyman radium capsules. Each capsule is loaded with 10 mg of radium. The capsules are inserted separately into the distended uterine cavity, using not less than six and not more than twelve (Figure 25). In this way it is claimed that a more homogeneous radiation distribution is delivered to the tumour mass. In addition to the Heyman capsules, ovoids are placed in the vaginal vault. The recommended dose is 4500 mg hours to the uterine cavity with an additional surface dose of 6000 rads to the vault of the vagina.

In Stage I cases, post-operative radium to the vault alone may be given. Various applicators have been described. The recommended dose is between 6000 and 7000 rads to the walls of the vagina.

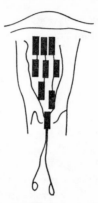

Figure 25   Heyman capsules

In more advanced disease, supplementary external radiation is recommended. One technique involves giving 4000 rads of megavoltage radiation in 4 to 5 weeks to the total pelvis. This is followed by a radium insertion of 2500 to 3000 mg hours. Two months later the patient may be scheduled for hysterectomy.

In very extensive disease, palliative radiotherapy can often relieve distressing symptoms for several years. This treatment may be augmented by progesterone therapy.

Results
Overall 5-year survival = 80 per cent.

The prognosis depends on the grade and stage of the tumour. Fortunately most cases are well-differentiated early Stage I lesions, with a uterine cavity of less than 8 cm. The 5-year survival for these patients treated by surgery and post-operative radium is better than 90 per cent.

In Stage III anaplastic lesions, the 5-year survival has dropped to 20 per cent with surgery alone. It is important to identify these patients in advance since their survival improves significantly with the more aggressive use of pre-operative radiation as described above.

VAGINA AND URETHRA
Squamous carcinoma of the vagina is a rare disease, sometimes associated with prolonged wearing of a pessary. Most tumours are sub-mucosal metastases

from adenocarcinoma of the endometrium. Metastases from the cervix, ovary and kidney are also seen. A tumour of Gartner's duct may sometimes occur. Sarcoma botryoides is discussed in Chapter 14.

Treatment

The primary lesions must be treated. This may call for surgical excision of the vagina and uterus by a vulval approach.

Superficial tumours of the upper third of the vagina may be treated by radium insertion as in carcinoma of the cervix but with the ovoids placed in tandem. Alternatively, a vaginal sorbo containing radium may be used.

Tumours of the anterior vagina and urethra are best treated by a gold seed or radium needle implant to a dose of 5500 rads in 7 days. More advanced tumours involving the base of bladder require external radiation to a dose of up to 7000 rads in 7 weeks. Suprapubic cystotomy and extended block dissection may also be required. However, surgical excision with transplantation of the ureters should only be considered in carefully selected patients in good general condition.

Tumours of the posterior wall of the vagina should be treated with a central radium source together with external radiation to the pelvic walls. A defunctioning colostomy is sometimes required before treatment.

CARCINOMA OF THE VULVA

This tumour is mostly found in elderly women and may be associated with leucoplakia. The histology is usually squamous carcinoma. Most lesions are on the anterior half of the vulva on the inner aspect of the labia near the clitoris. This may spread across the labia causing a 'kissing cancer' on the opposite side. Lymphatic drainage is rich and includes Cloquet's node in the femoral canal.

Treatment

The treatment of choice is radical vulvectomy leaving the vagina and urethra. The vulva is excised in continuity with the glands. Healing is by granulation, although a skin graft often helps recovery. The 5-year survival for operable cases is 70 per cent, but for those with involved lymph glands the prognosis is poor.

Vulval tumours are radioresistant. If surgery is contra-indicated, however, a radium or gold seed implant may be used. The rare tumour of the posterior third is best suited for an implant since surgery may damage the anal sphincter and cause incontinence. In this case it is important not to transfix the vagina or rectum during the implant, and a finger should be inserted in the rectum as a guide.

OVARIAN TUMOURS

The classification of ovarian tumours is difficult because although the majority are benign cystic swellings, a number of these merge into malignant disease. Most ovarian neoplasms are cystic carcinomas originating in epithelial tissue. The remainder are solid tumours, some of which are associated with endocrine features. No important aetiological factors have yet been identified.

Histology

1   Serous cystadenocarcinoma. This is the most common variety. It consists of ciliated columnar epithelium filled with serous fluid. These tumours may be papillary or multilocular. Fifty per cent of cases.

2   Pseudo-mucinous cystadenocarcinoma. This consists of columnar epithelium with mucinous vacuoles. The tumour may rupture leading to pseudomyxomata peritonei. It rarely metastasizes. Twelve per cent.

3   Unclassified solid adenocarcinoma. Varying degrees of de-differentiation are seen up to anaplastic carcinoma. Fifteen per cent.

4   Endometrioid adenocarcinoma. Fifteen per cent.

5   Malignant mesonephroma. Six per cent.

6   Granulosa cell tumour. This is potentially malignant. Divided into sarcomatoid and cylindroid or folliculoid types.

7   Thecoma. A feminizing tumour associated with carcinoma of the body of the uterus.

8   Arrhenoblastoma. Masculinizing tumour.

9   Dysgerminoma. The histological equivalent of seminoma of testes. Found in young women and associated with sexual maldevelopment.

10   Malignant teratoma.

11   Chorioncarcinoma.

Staging

Several different staging methods have been recommended. None is entirely satisfactory. The following system has been used in some hospitals and correlates with the results given below.

I   Confined to one ovary.

II   Invasion through capsule with microscopic lymph and blood spread. Accidental operative spillage. Both ovaries involved. Ascites with malignant cells in fluid.

III   (a) Infiltration of other pelvic viscera.
      (b) Intraperitoneal metastasis (not liver).

IV   Distant metastasis including liver.

Clinical Features

Unfortunately many ovarian tumours are silent in the early stages. Eventually pressure may produce pain, urinary frequency or torsion of the pedicle.

Endocrine symptoms may be the presenting feature. The tumour may also mimic pregnancy.

The six features of malignancy are:

1 Short history.
2 Ascites (50 per cent).
3 Bilateral swellings (50 per cent).
4 Sick facies.
5 Fixed swelling larger than an orange (5 cm).
6 Nodules in the cul-de-sac. (Pouch of Douglas.)

Investigations

1 Chest X-ray.
2 Intravenous pyelogram.
3 Endocrine assay where indicated.
4 Blood count.
5 Pelvic cytology.

Treatment

SURGERY. The diagnosis is usually only confirmed at laparotomy. At operation the surgeon should note specifically the extent of the disease, the presence of free fluid, peritoneal seeding or liver involvement. Peritoneal washings should be examined for the presence of malignant cells.

Most surgeons recommend pan-hysterectomy for all cases except those with advanced disease. Omentectomy appears to add little to survival. Conservative surgery may be sufficient if the lesion is well differentiated, encapsulated, single and pedunculated. In these cases the opposite ovary may sometimes be preserved in young women.

Residual disease following radiotherapy may occasionally be treated by further surgery, but exenteration is rarely indicated. A few tumours may be resectable at a second-look operation 6 weeks after radiotherapy. Since mucinous tumours rarely metastasize and are relatively radioresistant, some surgeons recommend a more aggressive surgical approach for these cases.

The granulosa cell tumour may recur up to 20 years after surgery. This happens more frequently in a sarcomatoid type, and radiotherapy is indicated for this tumour. In recurrent cylindroid tumours, pre-operative radiotherapy may facilitate removal of the lesion.

RADIATION THERAPY. Post-operative radiation therapy is recommended for most cases. In early disease, treatment may be confined to the pelvis. The recommended megavoltage dose for total pelvic irradiation is usually 4000 rads in 4 weeks.

In Stage III disease, total abdominal irradiation is recommended. This is better given through a moving-strip technique. In this way a dose of 3000 rads is delivered in 10 treatments to each strip (see Chapter 5).

Radiotherapy is of little curative value in Stage IV disease although useful palliation may be obtained by controlling large masses, reducing ascites and relieving pain.

If hysterectomy has not been performed, radium insertion may sometimes help, especially if the tumour is fixed in the true pelvis. The value of pre-operative radiation has not yet been fully assessed.

Dysgerminoma deserves special attention. This rare tumour is very radiosensitive. Surgical resection should be followed by an abdominal radiation bath shielding the kidneys. Most cases have lymphatic spread, and it may sometimes be necessary to treat the nodes above the diaphragm. A dose of 3000 rads in 3 weeks is usually adequate to control the disease.

Troublesome ascites may be treated by an intraperitoneal injection of 200 millicuries of radioactive colloidal gold 198 or radiophosphorus 32. Recently it has been shown that equally good results are obtained using alkylating agents.

CHEMOTHERAPY. The role of chemotherapy is still under investigation, and results are conflicting. Recently there has been renewed interest in the subject, and carefully controlled trials have been proposed.

Results

Overall 5-year survival = 30 per cent.
Stage I   = 75 per cent.
Stage II   = 60 per cent.
Stage III (a)   = 40 per cent.
Stage III (b)   = 15 per cent.
Stage IV   = 4 per cent.

Survival correlates more closely with stage than with histology, but unfortunately most cases present with advanced serous or undifferentiated carcinoma and consequently results are biased.

The best results are obtained with dysgerminoma where there is a 90 per cent survival.

CHORIONCARCINOMA

This is a unique tumour in that it is not derived from the host tissues but from the trophoblastic tissue of a parasite (foetus). The tumour is highly malignant and extremely rare. Sheets of polyhedral and giant cells invade the myometrium and spread rapidly by the bloodstream. Widespread haemorrhagic necrotic metastases occur. There are no normal chorionic villi.

Fifty per cent arise in hydatidiform moles, 25 per cent in abortions and 22 per cent in normal pregnancies. The remainder arise in ectopic pregnancies and in the ovaries.

Treatment

1 Surgery. For diagnosis. Some gynaecologists recommend total hysterectomy.

2 Chemotherapy. The drug of choice is the folic acid antagonist methotrexate. This can be combined with 6-mercaptopurine or an alkylating agent such as chlorambucil. Massive doses are recommended, and such treatment is best given in specialized isolated 'sterile islands' to prevent infection of the patient.

3 Radiotherapy. The tumour is radiosensitive but usually spreads too rapidly for effective control. Nevertheless a combination of radiotherapy to localized masses and chemotherapy may be useful in special cases.

4 Immunological therapy is under investigation.

Results

This is a remarkable tumour in that a large percentage of cases are cured by chemotherapy alone. Exact survival figures are unknown since the histological diagnosis can be difficult; normal trophoblastic tissue is invasive and may be confused with early lesions, making results appear better than they really are.

Chorioncarcinoma in the male has a bad prognosis. This is probably because there is no immunological rejection of the tumour in the male.

References

Allt, W. E. C. *Supervoltage radiation treatment in advanced cancer of the cervix*, Canad. Med. Assoc. J., 1969, **100**, 792.

Bagley, C. M., Young, R. C., Canelloa, G. P., and DeVita V. T. *Treatment of ovarian carcinoma*, New Eng. J. Med., 1972, **287**, 856.

Easson, E. C. *A comprehensive approach to cervical cancer*, Clin. Radiol., 1967, **18**, 337.

Fletcher, G. *Textbook of Radiotherapy*, Lea and Febiger, Philadelphia, 1973.

Ingersoll, F. B. *Vaginal recurrence of carcinoma of the corpus, Management and prevention*, Am. J. Surg., 1971, **121**, 473.

McGregor, E. *Carcinoma in situ*, Lancet, 1971, **1**, 74.

18

Male Genital Tract

TESTICULAR TUMOURS

Testicular cancer accounts for about 1 per cent of male cancer. The incidence appears to be rising, however. The reasons for this are not clear. Teratomas predominate at about 30 years of age and seminomas about 40 years. Thereafter the incidence declines but rises again around 70 years.

There is a definite association with undescended testes, but the effect of trauma or infection is unknown. The disease is more common in negroes.

Pathology

Seminoma is the only germinal tumour for which there is a generally accepted name. What we call 'teratoma' has always been confused by the need for names for the less-differentiated forms of this tumour. In the United States the term embryonal carcinoma is used to describe the anaplastic teratoma.

SEMINOMA. Seventy per cent of cases. This tumour arises in the germ cells. Histologically there are sheets of uniform large round cells with clear cytoplasm and central nuclei. There is a lymphocytic infiltration of the stroma, the intensity of which appears to be related to an immune response and a good prognosis.

TERATOMA. Twenty per cent of tumours. This disease probably arises in germ cells although there is some evidence that it represents abnormal development of toti-potential tissue. Squamous epithelium, cartilage, teeth and hair may be seen. One-third of teratomas contain seminomatous areas. Karyotyping of both tumours has confirmed marked aneuploidy.

MISCELLANEOUS TUMOURS. Interstitial Leydig cell tumours and Sertoli cell tumours are rarely malignant. Occasionally lymphomas of the testes have been reported. Chorioncarcinoma of the testes is extremely rare.

Spread

The tumour usually spreads by lymph channels along the spermatic vein to the para-aortic nodes. From there it may spread to the upper mediastinum and neck. There may also be retrograde spread to nodes at the brim of the pelvis. Blood spread may lead to 'cannon ball' metastases in the lungs and deposits in bone.

Clinical Features

Painless swelling with loss of sensation.
The right testis is often involved.
Clinically the testis feels heavy to the patient.
Gynaecomastia.
Metastatic features in nodes, bone and lungs.

Investigations

Chest X-ray.
Intravenous pyelogram.
Lymphangiogram.
Cavography.
Hormonal tests for urinary gonadotrophins.
Needle biopsy carries the risk of scrotal implantation and all suspicious swellings should be referred for surgery.

Treatment

SURGERY. Simple orchidectomy. The spermatic cord should be removed distal to the inguinal ring. The retroperitoneal tissue should not be disturbed, and lymph node dissection is not recommended. Radical orchidectomy with dissection of the retroperitoneal lymph nodes is widely practised for teratomas in the United States; in Britain the operation was virtually abandoned 20 years ago in favour of radiotherapy. There has, however, been some re-interest in laparotomy and lymph node biopsy for the purpose of surgically staging the disease.

RADIOTHERAPY. Seminomas are very radiosensitive. Even teratomas are more radiosensitive than was formerly thought.

Post-operative radiation should be given to all cases. The fields should include the regional lymph nodes, the para-aortic and the pelvic glands. Both kidneys should be protected. The recommended dose of mega-voltage radiation for seminomas lies between 2500 rads in 3 weeks and 3500 rads in 5 weeks. Higher doses — up to 5000 rads in 5 to 6 weeks — are suggested for teratomas. It is worth protecting the opposite testis since the incidence of bilateral tumour is less than 1·5 per cent. If this is done, the remaining gonad receives less than 100 rads and sterility may be avoided. Fields should be extended to include the mediastinum if it is involved. The value of prophylactic irradiation of the mediastinum and left supraclavicular fossa is unknown.

Metastases initially respond dramatically to radiation but often recur later. Rarely, patients with lung metastases have been controlled with small doses of radiation. This is usually combined with cytotoxic therapy, and a large number of drugs are currently under investigation.

Results

Seminoma: Overall 5-year survival = 65 per cent; for cases without metastases 80 per cent; with metastases 35 per cent.

Teratoma: Overall 5-year survival = 25 per cent; for cases without metastases 50 per cent; with metastases 10 per cent.

A bad prognosis is associated with long history, pain or gynaecomastia.

Complications

Following irradiation most patients develop some bowel reaction, but this usually clears. The high doses used for teratomas may lead to long-term intestinal damage in some patients. Radiation nephritis ensues if the kidney is not protected. Pulmonary fibrosis is inevitable if the dose to the lungs exceeds 2500 rads in 3 weeks.

CARCINOMA OF THE PENIS

This rare disease is usually only seen in the uncircumcized. It appears to be related to poor penile hygiene. In a large series reported from Jamaica, over half the patients had venereal disease. Thirty-five per cent of these cases had phimosis. The tumour is nearly always a squamous carcinoma.

Recently a case was reported in a patient whose wife had carcinoma of the cervix. Both patients had the same herpes antibodies in their sera.

Stage

- o   Intra-epithelial 'Erythroplasia of Queyrat'.
- I   Confined to penis.
- II   Mobile lymph nodes.
- III Fixed lymph nodes.

Treatment

Radiotherapy is recommended for early disease and for advanced cases with fixed inguinal glands. A dorsal slit is advisable in those patients presenting with phimosis. This permits the full extent of the lesion to be seen. It also allows the area to be kept clean during treatment and prevents troublesome oedema of the foreskin.

Patients may be treated by a box technique, the penis lying between two wax moulds with the fields applied to opposing sides. Orthovoltage or super-voltage radiation may be used. A dose of 4000 rads in 4 weeks to the shaft of the penis is often satisfactory. For superficial lesions, better cosmesis may be obtained using a cylindrical radium mould to a dose of 5500 rads in 7 days.

Queyrat's erythroplasia has been successfully treated with an yttrium 90 beta plaque. The suggested dose is 1500 rads in 10 minutes repeated after 1 week.

Amputation is recommended for lesions larger than 3 cm with invasion of the corpora and glans. Mobile lymph glands should be removed by surgical dissection. Pre-operative radiation is worthwhile in these patients. Advanced disease with fixed inguinal glands should be treated by radiation therapy. Although most of these cases are only suitable for palliation, an occasional patient may be salvaged with high dose irradiation.

Results

Five-year survival = 55 per cent.

The results of radiotherapy are as good as surgery in early cases and the advantages to the patient obvious. However, a few patients develop urethral stenosis following irradiation, and this may require frequent dilatation. Complications are more common with higher doses. Patients with fixed inguinal glands rarely survive but useful palliation may be obtained.

CARCINOMA OF THE SCROTUM

Mule spinners' cancer is no longer seen. However, there is today a clear-cut association between mineral oil and scrotal cancer in machine-tool setters.

The treatment of choice for early lesions is surgical excision. Unfortunately many patients delay seeking advice because of shyness. Advanced tumours may be treated by radiotherapy but this often results in sterility.

References

Annamunthodo, H. *Cancer of the penis*, Jour. Inter. Coll. Surg., 1961, **35**, 21.
Dayan, A., Blandy, J. P., and Hope-Stone, H. F. Symposium on Seminoma, Brit. J. Hosp. Med., 1966, November, 126.
Duncan, W., and Jackson, S. M. *The treatment of early cancer of the penis with megavoltage X-rays*, Clin. Radiol., 1972, **23**, 246.
Friedman, M. In *Treatment of Cancer and Allied Diseases*, ed. G. T. Pack and I. Ariel, Harper and Row, New York, 1964.
Maier, J. G., and van Buskirk. *Testicular malignancies*, J.A.M.A., 1970, **213**, 97.
Mantell, B. S., and Morgan, W. Y. *Erythroplasia of Querat*, Brit. J. Radiol., **42**, 855, 1969.

19

The Urinary Tract

HYPERNEPHROMA OF THE KIDNEY

This tumour usually arises in the tubules in the cortex of the upper pole of the kidney. A spherical yellow tumour may be found invading the renal vein and growing along it as a solid column of cells.

Histologically there are large vacuolated clear cells with pale cytoplasm in an acinar or papillary arrangement, interspaced with blood vessels. There may be retrograde emboli to the spermatic veins. Blood spread can lead to 'cannon ball' metastases in the lungs. Large painful pulsating bony metastases may also occur, especially in the humerus.

Clinical Features
1 Haematuria.
2 Loin pain.
3 Palpable abdominal mass.
4 Distant signs including varicocele, polycythaemia or metastatic lesions.

Investigations
1 Blood count.
2 Blood urea.
3 Urine analysis.
4 Chest X-ray.
5 Pyelogram. The calyces are thinned, elongated and spidery.
6 Aortograms and/or tomograms. These are usually essential for diagnosis. A tumour circulation (neovascularity) is seen in most cases.

Treatment
SURGERY. This is the treatment of choice.

RADIOTHERAPY. The place of radiation therapy in this disease is still uncertain. Post-operative radiation to the renal bed is usually recommended for advanced cases where there is lymphatic invasion, perinephric spread or incomplete removal of the tumour. Doses up to 4000 rads in 4 weeks are well tolerated. Anterior and posterior fields about 15 × 15 cm are usually required. The scar should be included in the field but the spinal cord wedged out if possible. The liver should also be shielded where possible.

Pre-operative radiation to a dose of 3000 rads may have a carcinostatic effect and at the same time shrink enlarged perinephric veins. Radiation may also shrink large inoperable tumours making surgery possible.

Results

Five-year survival = 35 per cent.

Some therapists claim that post-operative radiation therapy improves survival by a further 10 per cent.

The prognosis depends on the histological grade. Well-differentiated tumours have a better outlook than anaplastic tumours. Invasion of the renal vein is a bad prognostic sign.

Painful metastatic bone lesions may respond to palliative doses of radiotherapy.

Hypernephroma is an unusual tumour and metastatic lesions in the lung may remain unchanged in size for many years. A few single 'cannon ball' metastases have been successfully removed by lobectomy. Progesterone has been used with limited success in metastatic disease.

Wilm's Tumour

The reader is referred to Chapter 21 for a discussion of this tumour.

TUMOURS OF THE RENAL PELVIS

These are usually papillary transitional cell tumours and are often multicentric. Occasionally squamous metaplasia due to chronic irritation may lead to epidermoid carcinoma. Surgery is the treatment of choice, and post-operative radiation may be given if there has been incomplete excision or operative spill. A dose of 4000 to 5000 rads in 4 to 5 weeks is recommended.

CARCINOMA OF THE BLADDER

Aetiology

A number of aromatic amines have been implicated. These include naphthyl-amine, benzidine and the dyestuffs auramine and magenta. Aniline was formerly thought to be dangerous but is now known to be innocuous. Many of these chemicals have been used in the rubber and electric cable industries. Health officials believe that it is important to screen susceptible individuals for life, since tumours may develop up to 40 years following exposure. Occupational cancer of the bladder has also been found among rodent operatives using the chemical compound 'Antu'.

Other predisposing factors include polycythaemic patients treated with chlornaphazin, cigarette smoking and bilharziasis. Abnormalities of tryptophan metabolism may play an important role. There does not appear to be any connection between bladder stones and tumour formation, although stones may of course develop later.

Pathology

Many of these tumours probably start as benign papillomas which may be single or multiple. These may remain benign indefinitely or recur following removal. Eventually they may undergo malignant degeneration and extend locally through the wall of the bladder or give rise to distant metastases. Macroscopically the tumour may be papillary or solid, infiltrating or ulcerative.

Histologically, the lesion is usually a transitional cell carcinoma which may be well differentiated or anaplastic. More rarely, one may find squamous cell carcinoma, adenocarcinoma or sarcoma.

Stage

o   Benign papilloma.
I   Mucosa infiltration with intact basement membrane.
II   Muscularis invasion. Palpable induration bimanually.
III Extravesical but still mobile within the pelvis.
IV   Pelvic wall fixation or distant metastases.

Clinical Features

Cancer of the bladder is a disease of the elderly male. The triad of haematuria, increased urinary frequency and dysuria, singly or in combination, are the presenting features in 95 per cent of cases. The haematuria may be painless or accompanied by strangury.

Fifty per cent of tumours occur on the wall of the bladder, 20 per cent in the trigone, 10 per cent on the floor and 5 per cent on the roof. A further 5 per cent are multiple.

Investigations

1 Urine analysis and culture.
2 Chest X-ray and pyelogram. The latter is essential to rule out co-existing tumours of the renal pelvis or ureter.
3 Blood count.
4 Blood urea.
5 Cystogram.
6 Cystoscopy under anaesthesia. This is necessary both to locate the tumour and to obtain a biopsy specimen. An estimate of tumour size can be made by comparing it to the distance between the ureteric orifices, which is about 4 cm. A good bimanual examination can only be achieved under anaesthesia when the bladder is empty and relaxed. At the same time it is important to rule out a double primary of the rectum, cervix or prostate.

Treatment

General measures are essential and all patients should be given prophylactic urinary antibiotics. A few require blood transfusion. The treatment policy must then consider two main aspects:

1 The depth of infiltration and the risk of lymph node involvement.
2 The multifocal extent of the lesion which may include the rest of the urinary tract.

DIATHERMY. Stage 0 and Stage I lesions may be controlled for many years by cystoscopic resection or coagulation with deep diathermy.

PARTIAL CYSTECTOMY. This should be reserved for vault tumours or small tumours near the ureteric orifice where it is possible to excise the lesion and anastomose the ureter. Elsewhere this treatment should not be used unless the tumour is single and small with a sharp margin. Areas of 'mossy' mucosa or multiple lesions should not be treated in this way.

RADIOTHERAPY. Currently this is the treatment of choice for deeply infiltrating Stage II, III or IV lesions. Supervoltage radiation is required. Radical doses of up to 6000 rads in 6 weeks are recommended. A multiple field or rotation technique should be used to protect the rectum as much as possible.

A cystogram is essential to locate the tumour site. The fields are usually centred on a treatment volume of about $9 \times 9 \times 9$ cm. Most therapists treat the whole bladder, or even the whole pelvis, especially where there is extensive involvement of the mucous membrane. However, radiation tolerance depends on the volume of tissue treated, and the field sizes should be kept as small as possible above doses of 4000 rads.

Recurrences in surgical scars are common, and the dose to the skin should be built up in such areas.

RADIOACTIVE ISOTOPES. Radioactive isotopes are now used less often in the treatment of bladder cancer. Some therapists recommend a radon or gold seed implant to a dose of 5000 rads for localized (4×4 cm maximum) Stage I or II lesions. This can be followed by a dose of 4000 rads external radiation to the whole bladder.

Tantalum 182 wire bent into 'hairpins' can be implanted into the bladder wall. Attached threads enable the wire to be removed through the urethra after 1 week. A dose of 7000 rads in 7 days is suggested. Implants are best done at open operation since it is difficult to obtain good geometry using the trans-urethral route. Tantalum wire has also been used to prevent 'seeding' in scars.

Results with balloons containing radioactive Cobalt 60 beads have not been entirely satisfactory.

Other radioactive isotopes used include intracavitary installation of colloidal gold 198 or yttrium 90. These are said to prevent 'seeding' prior to open operation. Installation of thiotepa has also been recommended for the same purpose.

RADICAL SURGERY. Total cystectomy is indicated for recurrence following radiotherapy or for severe radiation sequelae. It is also the treatment of choice for multiple lesions involving the ureter or urethra. Many of these tumours are well-differentiated papillary lesions and are radioresistant. Patients should obviously be in good general condition before major surgery is considered since the operation carries an appreciable mortality. Following surgery there is the problem of urinary diversion, either to the isolated rectum which leaves the patient with a colostomy, or to a colonic or ileal conduit. These patients may subsequently develop pyelonephritis. There is also the problem of chloride re-absorption and hyperchloremic acidosis although this can usually be controlled with sodium bicarbonate.

Many patients with advanced tumours treated by radiotherapy die from local disease in the pelvis without evidence of distant metastases. These radiation failures may be due to unfavourable tumour bed produced by infection and anoxia. Among suggestions for improving results are the surgical relief of any urinary obstruction, urinary diversion, neutron therapy and high pressure oxygen irradiation. More aggressive treatment with pre-operative irradiation followed by radical surgery has also been recommended in selected cases.

Results

The survival figures for early disease are confusing. This is mainly because there is no clear-cut border between benign and malignant disease. However the following 5-year survival results are quoted:

Stage I   = 80 per cent.
Stage II   = 57 per cent.
Stage III = 31 per cent.
Stage IV   = 10 per cent.

Well-differentiated papillary lesions have a better prognosis than solid anaplastic tumours.

Relief of symptoms is often dramatic following small doses of radiation. Dysuria and distressing haematuria may clear following doses of about 2500 rads.

Complications

Post-radiation haemorrhagic cystitis.
Telangiectasia of the bladder.
Contracted bladder.

Urinary tract complications terminating with uraemia.
Bowel disturbance with fistula formation.
Perineal fibrosis.

CARCINOMA OF THE PROSTATE

Histologically 'latent' cancer is found in the prostate glands of 75 per cent of elderly men. However, only a small proportion of these cases develop clinical evidence of prostatic carcinoma. The disease is rare below 50 years.

The prostate is a retroperitoneal gland with three lobes. Carcinoma most often involves the posterior lobe. The lesion is usually an adeno-carcinoma. It has a well-defined tubular pattern of uniform cuboidal cells with small dark central nuclei and clear cytoplasm. Various degrees of de-differentiation are seen. Eventually the tumour breaks through the capsule and invades vessels and perineural lymphatics. It may then spread directly to the periprostatic tissue or give rise to distant bony metastases.

Stage

I   Occult tumour not palpable rectally.
II   Confined within prostatic capsule. Palpable rectally.
III Local extension or enzyme elevation.
IV   Extra-pelvic disease.

Clinical Features

The patient may present with urinary symptoms identical to those of benign enlargement of the prostate. There may be symptoms of metastatic deposits, particularly low back pain.

Rectal palpation provides the diagnosis in about 50 per cent of cases; enlargement of the posterior lobe replaces the normal sulcus between the lateral lobes with a hard craggy mass.

The serum acid phosphatase is raised above 4 K.A. units in half of the cases.

About one quarter of the patients have X-ray evidence of metastatic bony deposits which are usually osteosclerotic. These can sometimes be confused with Paget's disease.

A biopsy should be obtained where possible. This may be done via the trans-urethral route although occasionally an open biopsy through the perineum may be necessary.

Treatment

RADIOTHERAPY. There is an increasing trend towards the use of high dose external radiotherapy to treat this disease, especially in those patients whose prostatic cancer is already invasive. It has been difficult to evaluate this modality because the natural history of the disease is not yet fully understood.

However, even in those patients whose disease course seems to be inexorable, radiation appears to improve both the length of survival and quality of life.

Radiotherapy is indicated in young men with aggressive anaplastic lesions. These patients often have a low acid phosphatase and usually do not respond to hormone therapy.

Several series of cases have now been treated with supervoltage radiation. The best responses have been obtained where the tumour is confined to the prostate, its capsule or the periprostatic tissue. Doses of up to 7000 rads in 6 weeks have been recommended. The tumour can be localized radiographically using a Foley catheter, with a small amount of mercury to outline the bladder base. The lower edge of the anterior field is defined 1 cm below the pubic margin and the posterior field 1 cm below the anus. The treatment field sizes usually vary between 6×6 cm and 12×12 cm, depending on the extent of the disease. The final part of treatment can be given by rotation therapy.

Extended field radiotherapy has also been recommended, especially in the more advanced stages. In these cases spread to the pelvic lymph nodes is common, and this may be demonstrated on lymphangiography. One technique calls for irradiation of the pelvic lymph nodes to a dose of 4800 rads followed by an additional 2400 rads to the prostate itself. This high dose has to be extended over an 11-week period.

Interstitial radioactive implants had a brief vogue in the treatment of prostatic cancer but the technique is still under investigation and has not been widely adopted.

Radiotherapy may also provide relief of painful metastatic bone lesions.

SURGERY. The results of surgery are disappointing, but radical prostatectomy still has a limited place in the treatment of a few selected early cases. The operation usually causes impotence. The role of surgery in staging the disease may become increasingly important again. Retropubic exploration permits extensive lymph node biopsy and, in one large series, has produced little morbidity and no mortality.

HORMONE THERAPY. Many cases of prostatic carcinoma are androgen dependent. For this reason, hormonal therapy and orchidectomy are sometimes recommended. Following castration, 70 per cent of patients have a temporary remission and 10 per cent a prolonged response. Hormonal therapy is especially recommended for advanced cases. Stilboestrol has been prescribed in varying dose schedules ranging from 1 mg daily up to 100 mg daily. Better results have been claimed using the phosphate ester of Stilboestrol, 'Honvan'. This drug is activated by the enzyme prostatic acid phosphatase and is alleged to release Stilboestrol locally, giving high concentrations in the tumour.

Hypophysectomy and adrenalectomy have occasionally been recommended as a last resort in advanced disease. Occasional remissions have also been obtained with Progesterone.

Results

Prolonged cures are now being claimed for high dose radiation therapy for invasive carcinoma. In one series, a 5-year survival of 60 per cent is quoted for combined stage II and III disease and a 10-year survival of 40 per cent.

Bladder invasion is an ominous finding. In a series of 13 patients with biopsy-proven bladder involvement, only one patient was living and free from disease three years following therapy.

Oestrogen therapy has a number of disturbing side effects including nausea, fluid retention and gynaecomastia. Caution is advised in the presence of cardiovascular disease. In a widely quoted series of patients treated with hormones at the Veterans' Administration Hospitals in the United States, equivocal results have been obtained. This is in contrast to the experience of most urologists who report that the symptomatic improvement following hormonal therapy is enormous. It may be, however, that the VA patient population is a highly selected group with possible concomitant liver and cardiac disease. Even so, it is doubtful if androgen withdrawal actually prolongs life although it produces obvious relief of symptoms in many cases.

Gynaecomastia can be prevented by giving a course of superficial radiation to the breast tissue prior to hormonal administration. The recommended dose is 900 rads in three treatments on alternate days.

References

Bloedorn, F. G. *Carcinoma of the bladder*, in *Textbook of Radiotherapy*, ed. G. Fletcher, Lea and Febiger, Philadelphia, 1966.
Frank, H. G. *Treatment of carcinoma of bladder by radiotherapy*, Clin. Radiol., 1970, **21**, 425.
Symposium on prostatic cancer, Hospital Practice, 1972, January, 41.

20

Breast

Breast cancer is the commonest form of female cancer in Europe and North America. Seven per cent of all women contract the disease. Despite recent advances in treatment, the mortality has remained almost unchanged during the past 30 years.

AETIOLOGY OF BREAST CARCINOMA

The cause of breast carcinoma remains obscure, but a number of pre-disposing factors have been established by statistical analysis.

AGE. The disease is virtually unknown in women under 20 years.

HORMONAL FACTORS. Single women are more liable to develop breast cancer. On the other hand, increasing parity beyond two children has a protective effect. Breast-feeding is not an important protective mechanism except in extensive and prolonged feeding.

Investigations have shown that urinary androgen metabolite excretion is subnormal in about half of the patients. Statistics also indicate that early menarche and late menopause are associated with an increased incidence of breast cancer.

DIET. There is some evidence that excessive oil and fat intake increases the risk.

RADIATION. This is a rare but well-recognized cause.

HEREDITY. This is not a major factor but is involved in some cases. Women whose mothers or sisters have had breast cancer have a twice normal incidence.

PRE-EXISTING DISEASE. There is an association with chronic cystic mastitis but not with fibro-adenomata. There also seems to be a relationship with tumours of the salivary gland.

PATHOLOGY

Histology

1. INFILTRATING CARCINOMA. (*a*) Schirrous duct. This is the most common variety (70 per cent of cases) and is divided into spheroidal, polyhedral and cuboidal cell types. (*b*) Medullary. Spheroidal cells with lymphoid stroma. Seven per cent of cases. (*c*) Rare types include squamous metaplasia, mucoid (colloid), intracystic papillary type and cylindroma. Seven per cent of cases.

2. NON-INFILTRATING CARCINOMA (carcinoma-in-situ). (*a*) Paget's — epidermal. One per cent of cases. (*b*) Comedocarcinoma. Intra-duct type. Four per cent of cases. (*c*) Intralobular. Five per cent of cases but may be higher.

Spread

The disease spreads directly through the chest wall and along lymph channels. Blood spread with distant metastases can occur at any stage.

Lymph Drainage

This follows the blood supply:

1. Along the perforating branches of internal mammary vessels which pierce each intercostal space, to nodes on the internal mammary chain. These nodes are also supplied from the lateral perforating branches of intercostal vessels. They are involved in 30 per cent of cases.

2. To the axilla, supra-clavicular nodes, sub-clavian node and thoracic duct on the left.

The axillary nodes are (*a*) anterior — deep to pectoralis major; (*b*) posterior — along sub-scapular vessels; (*c*) lateral — along axillary vein; (*d*) central — in axillary fat; (*e*) apical — from all other nodes.

Deposits can block pathways and retrograde spread may then occur to the opposite breast, groin, internal mammary chain and the neck. Supra-clavicular involvement is always associated with axillary involvement.

Stage

The TNM method is widely used (see page 40).
T_1 — Tumour under 2 cms. T_2 — over 2 cms. T_3 — skin infiltration or chest wall attachment.
N_0 — No nodes. N_1 — mobile nodes. N_2 — fixed nodes.
M_0 — No distant metastases. M_1 — distant metastases.

Many clinicians feel that conventional methods of staging should be abandoned and replaced by a more intensive search for metastatic disease when the patient is first seen.

Clinical Features

Most patients present with a painless lump in the breast. Occasionally there is bleeding from the nipple or frank ulceration of the skin. Some cases present with metastatic disease, and a close search may be required before the primary lesion is found.

INVESTIGATIONS

1. BIOPSY. Fine needle aspiration is usually satisfactory for diagnosis but all suspicious lumps should be removed if there is any doubt. It is worth recalling the aphorism, 'no lady should have a lump in her breast.'

2. MAMMOGRAM. This is a positive test in 90 per cent of the cases and may detect a tumour up to 4 years before it is clinically palpable.

3. X-RAYS. Chest, skull, spine and pelvis. Spinal metastases usually cause pain and are often not seen on X-ray in the early stages.

4. BONE SCAN. This is the most promising investigation at the present time. It often detects metastases not visible on X-ray.

5. THERMOGRAPHY. This investigation is still in the experimental stage but is useful in experienced hands.

TREATMENT

This is probably the most controversial subject in cancer therapy today. Before discussing the choice of therapy, the two main alternatives are presented.

Surgery

Surgery may be limited to biopsy excision or 'lumpectomy'. Simple mastectomy comprises removal of the breast. In extended simple mastectomy several axillary lymph nodes are also removed. Radical mastectomy consists of removing the breast plus 5 cm of skin around the nipple, the pectoralis major and minor muscles, the axillary fat and nodes and the sub-clavian nodes. The operation can be extended to include the parasternal chain by removing the 2nd, 3rd and 4th rib cartilages and sternal border. Dissection of the supra-clavicular fossa has been virtually abandoned since this is the third level of involvement. In the modified radical mastectomy, the pectoralis is left undisturbed, but there is a full dissection of axillary nodes. In medial quadrant tumours, biopsy of the internal mammary node may be helpful in planning subsequent treatment.

Radiotherapy

Post-operative radiation may be given to the chest wall and lymph node drainage areas. Several modifications of the following plan have been used.

Two opposed glancing fields about 10 × 15 cm are directed tangentially across the chest wall through the scar on the affected side (Figure 26a and b).

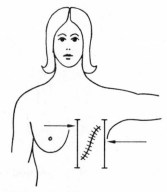

Figure 26a   Superficial glancing chest wall fields

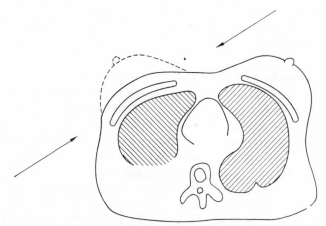

Figure 26b   Cross-sectional view of glancing fields

The parasternal and supra-clavicular nodes can be irradiated through an inverted L-shaped field (Figure 27). The axilla may be included in this arrangement. A posterior portal may be used to boost the dose to the axilla and supra-clavicular fossa if necessary. Supervoltage therapy is preferable for the lymph node areas, but orthovoltage radiation is adequate for the chest wall. Compensating filters may be used to adjust the variation in dosimetry over the sterno-clavicular contours. A dose of 4500 rads in 3 weeks is probably sufficient, although higher doses have also been advocated.

Radiation may be the primary mode of treatment in breast cancer. In this case, a modification of the above technique is used and somewhat higher doses, up to 5500 rads in 5 weeks, are recommended.

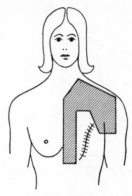

Figure 27   Direct irradiation of lymph node drainage region

The Choice of Therapy

In view of the variety of surgical and radiotherapeutic techniques, it is not surprising that there is some statistical confusion about results. The need for prospective controlled clinical trials has been recognized, and these are now under way in many centres. Meanwhile the results of three separate trials are available.

In the Manchester trial, radical mastectomy followed by post-operative radiotherapy was compared with radical mastectomy alone. The latter group received radiotherapy only if subsequent local recurrence of cancer developed. The survival rates in both groups were comparable after 10 years.

In the Cambridge trial, simple mastectomy plus radiotherapy was compared with radical mastectomy plus radiotherapy. The results were similar in both groups. Indeed, if anything, the simpler procedure was better.

The Copenhagen trial compared simple mastectomy plus radiotherapy with extended radical mastectomy. Once again there was no difference in survival in the two groups. There was, however, a higher morbidity following extended mastectomy.

It seems likely that the die is cast when the patient first visits her physician. At that moment, distant disease may already be present. Thus the eventual outcome is probably predetermined regardless of the local treatment. Biopsy excision of the lump combined with adequate radiotherapy may yield equally good results at all stages. However, such treatment necessitates close follow-up, and it is often difficult to know whether subsequent local thickening in the treated area represents recurrence or radiation fibrosis. Many patients sense the physician's uncertainty and would have preferred simple mastectomy in the first instance.

It is impossible to obtain general agreement on the best form of therapy. In Britain, simple mastectomy followed by radiotherapy is now advocated by almost half of the surgeons. In the USA radical mastectomy is still practised in most hospitals. Two alternative treatment plans are presented below:

PLAN A. *Early disease:* Simple mastectomy followed by a full course of radiation therapy. The rationale for this is as follow:

1. Results appear to be as good as radical mastectomy with or without radiotherapy.
2. It avoids the morbidity of radical mastectomy where an appreciable number of patients develop lymphoedema of the upper limb.
3. It prevents chest wall recurrence.
4. Parasternal disease may be arrested.

Late disease: Local radiotherapy. Chemotherapy.

PLAN B. *Early disease*: Modified radical mastectomy. Post-operative radiotherapy is given only if there is histological evidence of spread of disease.

Late disease: The primary lesion may be controlled with local surgery or radiotherapy. Chemotherapy may then be given when the patient develops active disease elsewhere.

METASTATIC DISEASE

Radiotherapy
Painful bony metastases may be treated by radiation. Relief is often dramatic. Metastases in the skin, orbit and brain may also be treated with small palliative doses of radiation. Small recurrent nodules on the chest wall can often be re-treated even if the area has been previously irradiated.

Endocrine Therapy and Chemotherapy
Once disseminated disease causes symptoms the following steps may be taken, although not necessarily in the order given.

1. Ovarian ablation (by radiation or surgery) to pre-menopausal patients and those within 5 years of the menopause. About 30 per cent obtain some benefit, and in about half of these the remission is really worthwhile.

2. Androgens may be given to the above group of patients. About 20 per cent respond. 25 to 50 mg testosterone propionate intramuscularly is a suitable compound to use. The inevitable virilization and altered libido are often unacceptable to patients and consequently relatively non-virilizing androgens are being developed.

3. Oestrogens are recommended for patients more than 5 years post-menopausal. The older the patient, the better the remission; 60 per cent of

the cases over 70 years obtain a worthwhile response. Ethinyloestradiol is usually given at a dosage 0·5 mg t.d.s. Nausea can be avoided if treatment is started gradually. Withdrawal vaginal bleeding occurs if treatment is stopped abruptly.

4. Progestogens may produce remissions in a few cases. Anti-oestrogenic hormonal therapy may also be tried.

5. Corticosteroid therapy is often beneficial, even in the absence of a previous response to other measures.

6. Adrenalectomy or hypophysectomy should be considered if and when hormonal therapy fails. The best results are obtained where hypophysectomy is complete.

7. Cytotoxic therapy: Cyclophosphamide and vincristine have both been used. More recently combination drug programmes have been developed with encouraging results. (See chemotherapy, Chapter 24.)

In considering the above regimens it is important to note that a remission of withdrawal may sometimes follow cessation of a drug.

Biochemical and clinical guides have been devised to identify suitable patients before subjecting them to hypophysectomy. There is as yet no general agreement about results. However, studies of growth hormone levels and prolactin metabolism may be helpful in detecting hormonal-dependent tumours.

PROGNOSIS

Overall 5-year survival = 45 per cent.
Overall 10-year survival = 33 per cent.
Overall 15-year survival = 20 per cent.

Stages I and II
5-year survival = 60 per cent.
10-year survival = 39 per cent.
15-year survival = 35 per cent.

Breast cancer in the early stages appears to be a curable disease. After 12 years, the survival curve for these cases follows that of the general population. The failures in this group probably had metastases when first seen.

Stages III and IV
5-year survival = 17 per cent.
10-year survival = 4 per cent.

Twenty per cent of all patients have obvious advanced disease when first seen. By definition, most of these cases are incurable but a few with slow-growing tumours survive for long periods of time. A further 50 per cent of patients probably have occult metastases when first seen. The remainder of cases are potentially curable.

Following surgery alone, local recurrence will develop in up to 25 per cent of patients. Most of these cases also have distant disease, but a few, 4 per cent, have pure recurrence. Post-operative radiotherapy prevents local recurrence, although results seem equally good if irradiation is withheld until the time of recurrence.

Very rarely, local recurrence develops in the irradiated area. Some clinicians have suggested that this unusual picture is due to radiation-induced immunoparesis. Others believe that it is due to blockage of lymphatic vessels coupled with an inadequate dose and point out that further radiation treatment often eradicates the disease.

Infiltration of the axillary nodes has a profound effect on prognosis. The greater the number of affected nodes, the greater the mortality. Furthermore, there is good evidence that when the disease spreads above the lower border of the pectoralis minor muscle, it is incurable.

The length of history, histological grade and anatomical site are thought to influence prognosis but the relationships are complex. It has been shown, however, that medullary carcinoma has a much better prognosis than schirrous carcinoma.

Care should be taken to examine the opposite breast at follow-up since this is a frequent site for metastases. Furthermore, breast cancer patients are more liable than the normal population to develop a second primary.

CANCER OF THE MALE BREAST

This condition is extremely rare probably because of the scant male mammary tissue and perhaps also because of hormonal factors. The disease has a bad prognosis because this lack of tissue leads to early chest wall fixation.

Orchidectomy is indicated for advanced cases. The remission rate is about 65 per cent and the duration of remission much longer than that for female breast cancer.

References

Atkins, H., Hayward, J. L., Klugman, D. J., and Wayte, A. B. *Treatment of Early Breast Cancer*, Brit. Med. J., 1972, **2**, 243.

British Medical Journal, Editorial, 1970, 7 March, 579.

Conservative treatment of breast cancer, Proc. Inter. Conference, Strasbourg, 1972 (in press).

Forrest, A. P. M., Burn, J., and Hayward, J. *Current practice: Cancer of the breast*, Brit. Med. J., 1970, **2**, 465.

Garrett, M. J. Clin. Radiol., 1969, **20**, 110.

Stoll, Basil A. *Hormonal management of advanced breast cancer*, Brit. Med. J. 1969, **2**, 293.

Symposium on Breast Cancer, Cancer, 1971, **28**, 6.

21

Malignant Disease in Childhood and Pregnancy

The commonest form of malignant disease in young people is acute leukaemia (see Chapter 16). The solid tumours of childhood are mainly undifferentiated lesions arising in embryonic mesoderm. These include Wilm's tumour, neuroblastoma and medulloblastoma. Most of these lesions are highly radiosensitive. However, normal tissue grows rapidly in childhood and is also radiosensitive. This is particularly true of brain tissue and the epiphyses of growing bones. Unlike adults, children have active marrow in their long bones which assists recovery from extensive radiation treatment.

Tissue Tolerance
The following limits of radiation tolerance have been reported in children: 3000 rads in 6 weeks to a 20 cm length of spinal cord; 4000 rads in 6 weeks to the whole brain; 1500 rads in 4 weeks to both lung fields, and 1200 rads in 2 weeks to the kidney.

Bone growth will be stunted if the dose exceeds 2000 rads in 2 weeks. If a hemivertebra is irradiated, it may result in wedging and scoliosis, although whole vertebra irradiation does not necessarily prevent this. The lens of the eye is very sensitive in children. It should be shielded where possible since radiation cataracts do badly in young people. It is also important to protect the endocrine and reproductive glands.

General Approach
Although children do not usually appreciate the prognosis, they should be treated with confidence and warmth. It is better to use tact and understanding, but if very young patients refuse to lie still on the treatment table they should not be restrained forcibly. If anaesthesia is required, rectal pentothal is recommended. Finally, one must remember that follow-up for life although theoretically desirable is hardly feasible.

NEPHROBLASTOMA (WILM'S TUMOUR)

This tumour arises from abnormal differentiation of embryonic renal tissue. Histologically there are mixed epidermal and mesodermal elements including cartilage and muscle fibres. The embryonic epithelial cells are often arranged in rosettes and contain formed and abortive renal elements. The supporting connective tissue of spindle cells is also malignant.

The spread is opposite to that already described for hypernephroma (Chapter 19). At first there is local invasion. Lymph and blood-borne metastases appear late. Malignant cells eventually spread to the renal vein, inferior vena cava, the opposite renal vein and the right atrium to the lungs.

A sub-group — mesoblastic nephroma — has been recognized. This lesion seems to be of low-grade malignancy, if not benign, and may contribute to the recognized better survival in infants. Wilm's tumour has occurred *in utero* but is usually found between 15 months and 3 years. There have been rare cases in older children and even adults. The disease may be associated with congenital malformations such as aniridia, hemihypertrophy and hypospadias. Approximately 5 per cent of Wilm's tumours occur in a solitary kidney (congenital absence) or horseshoe kidney. Ten per cent of cases are bilateral.

Clinical Features
The tumour may present with haematuria, urinary tract symptoms or an abdominal mass with constitutional upset. Hypertension has occasionally been noted and is associated with a poor prognosis. Rarely polycythaemia may be found.

Investigations
1 Straight X-ray abdomen: Curvilinear 'egg shell' calcification is sometimes seen in contrast to the amorphous calcification of neuroblastoma.
2 Intravenous pyelogram: Wilm's tumour rarely crosses the midline but deviation of a ureter may denote extension to para-aortic nodes.
3 Inferior vena cavagram: A better outline of the tumour may be obtained if cavagram is combined with pyelogram.
4 Chest X-ray: The lungs are the commonest site for metastases. Careful evaluation of the chest in both obliquities is necessary. Laminograms may be required.

Treatment

1. SURGERY. Nephrectomy is advised as soon as possible. The surgical findings are a prognostic guide and should be noted carefully. The important points to look for are fixation of the tumour, lymph node involvement and tumour in the capsular and renal veins. The other kidney should always be examined. Metallic clips can be used to denote the margins of extension. The ovaries may occasionally be re-implanted outside the proposed radiation fields.

If the tumour is too large to be removed it can often be rendered operable by a course of radiotherapy.

2. RADIOTHERAPY. Wilm's tumour is highly radiosensitive, and post-operative radiation is recommended for all cases. Occasionally in infants under 1 year, if the tumour is well differentiated and entirely confined to its capsule, surgery alone may suffice.

Medium voltage radiotherapy is satisfactory, but megavoltage gives less bone absorption and a more homogeneous radiation distribution. Anterior and posterior fields should be directed to the tumour bed and adjacent para-aortic nodes. The limits are usually the diaphragm above and the inferior mesenteric artery below. Massive tumours may require fields stretching from the nipple line to the pelvic floor. The femoral epiphysis, iliac crests and opposite kidney should be shielded where possible.

The dose is scaled according to age, ranging from 2500 rads for young children to 3500 rads and above for older children. If larger fields are required the dose may have to be reduced slightly. Treatment should start at about 50 rads per day and then gradually be increased to 150 rads per day.

A few cases of lung metastases have responded to pulmonary irradiation, but the dose must be kept below 2000 rads in 4 weeks to prevent pulmonary fibrosis and cor pulmonale.

3. CHEMOTHERAPY. Actinomycin D in a dose up to 120 mcg/kg by daily injection for 1 week is recommended if metastases are suspected. A 2-year course of prophylactic actinomycin D has been recommended for all older children, but the exact role of chemotherapy is still under investigation.

Other forms of chemotherapy under trial include cyclophosphamide, daunomycin and vincristine.

Results
Five-year survival = 30 per cent.

Better results are quoted with the combined approach of surgery, radiotherapy and chemotherapy, but these results have not yet been fully confirmed. There is no doubt, however, that infants have a better prognosis than older children.

Those patients who develop lung metastases usually do so inside 1 year. Cases surviving 3 years, or who double their age from conception, rarely have recurrence. Some morbidity is occasionally inevitable, and patients may be left with stunted growth and amenorrhoea. A few late cases of second primary tumours induced by radiation have been reported.

NEUROBLASTOMA

This tumour arises in neuroectoderm. Most cases originate in the adrenal medulla, but the disease may be found anywhere in the sympathetic chain from the nasopharynx (organ of Jacobson) to the pelvis (organ of Zuckerkandl). Older children tend to get a more differentiated form of tumour, the ganglio-neuroma. This lesion can be considered a juvenile form of phaeochromo-cytoma.

Neuroblastoma usually presents as an abdominal mass in infants under 1 year. In older children metastatic bone pain is a common feature. The disease also metastasizes to the liver (Peppard's syndrome) and to the skull and orbit (Hutchinson's syndrome). Peri-orbital ecchymosis in the absence of trauma is almost pathognomonic for neuroblastoma at any age. Mediastinal adenopathy usually represents evidence of extension, but lung parenchymal metastases are uncommon (unlike Wilm's tumour).

Investigations
Full radiographic survey of the skeleton is essential. Calcification of the primary occurs in 25 per cent of cases. Metastases do not usually calcify, and if liver calcification is seen, it is often due to a primary hepatic tumour.

Bone marrow biopsy is essential. It may be positive before radiographic changes are evident.

Biochemical tests of urinary catecholamines have added to the accuracy of diagnosis. They allow evaluation of progress and control of the disease and may detect early recurrence. Both homovanillic acid (HVA) and vanila-mandelic acid (VMA) are raised in the disease. Cystotheionine estimation is also of value and is raised in the more malignant and metastasizing forms of neuroblastoma.

Treatment
Surgical exploration is necessary for biopsy and confirmation of the diagnosis. It is most unusual to find a well-encapsulated lesion. If the tumour cannot be completely removed, the margins of residual disease should be marked with metallic clips. An attempt may occasionally be made to salvage the kidney. If it is not involved it may sometimes be repositioned safely outside the radiation field.

The tumour is highly radiosensitive, and radiotherapy to the tumour bed is advised for most cases. The technique is similar to that for Wilm's tumour. The recommended dose lies between 2000 and 3000 rads in 2 to 4 weeks. In infants under 1 year a dose of 1200 rads is often sufficient. Indeed doses as low as 800 rads in five treatments have resulted in permanent cures in some patients.

For palliative purposes, 450 rads in 3 days will often give marked pain relief and regression of disfiguring masses. Higher doses of 1500 to 2000 rads in 2 weeks may be needed to control intracranial and scalp metastases.

Chemotherapy plays a vital part in the management of neuroblastoma. Nitrogen mustard, cyclophosphamide and vincristine have been used in combination and in addition to radiation. Bone marrow involvement is an absolute indication for chemotherapy. The question of how long drug therapy should be continued, especially in infants, is still being investigated.

Prognosis

In assessing results, it must be remembered that neuroblastoma has the highest rate of spontaneous regression of any known tumour (up to 8 per cent of cases). Survival depends more on age than on the extent of the disease. A 2-year survival without recurrence represents a cure in most cases. For infants under 1 year the 2-year survival is 75 per cent; for older children the 2-year survival is 20 per cent. The overall 2-year survival is 35 per cent. Cases with localized disease in the mediastinum have the best prognosis and those with retroperitoneal or primary adrenal tumours a bad prognosis. Bone involvement is nearly always fatal. On the other hand, the improved prognosis reported in infants holds even in the presence of liver metastases. This has been noted in several other embryonic tumours of childhood and may be related to passive immunological factors.

MISCELLANEOUS TUMOURS

Ninety per cent of brain tumours in children under 5 years are in the cerebellar fossa. Most of these growths are well-differentiated astrocytomas and respond well to surgery. Occasionally ependymoblastoma has been reported. Medulloblastoma, haemangioblastoma and retinoblastoma have already been discussed.

Malignant lymphomas are relatively common in young people. These are discussed in Chapter 15.

Other rare tumours that respond to radiotherapy include sarcoma botryoides (rhabdomyosarcoma), the mesonephroma of the ovary and the juvenile angiofibroma of the nasopharynx. Osteogenic sarcoma usually occurs in young people in their late teens. The disease is discussed under bone tumours (Chapter 14).

MALIGNANT DISEASE IN PREGNANCY

The teratogenic properties of radiation are well known. Thus the management of cancer in pregnancy presents special problems.

The disease process is often more advanced for two reasons: firstly, diagnosis may be delayed because both patient and doctor attribute early symptoms to pregnancy; secondly, the increased blood volume and metabolic rate in pregnancy can lead to early metastases.

Breast Cancer

The co-existence of breast cancer and pregnancy is frequently regarded as sinister. Yet surveys indicate that a poor prognosis is associated only with cancer that is diagnosed and treated during the second half of pregnancy.

Patients in whom treatment was delayed until after delivery fared much better.

It is recommended that if breast cancer develops in the first half of pregnancy, it should be treated by orthodox methods and the pregnancy need not be terminated. If radiotherapy is involved, the dose to the foetus will probably not greatly exceed that used in diagnostic procedures. Tumours appearing in late pregnancy should have treatment delayed until after delivery. This may be induced once the foetus is viable.

Pregnancy occurring after primary treatment of breast cancer does not worsen prognosis. In fact, if anything the 10-year survival rate is slightly higher.

Carcinoma of the Cervix

The most vital point in treatment is to avoid delivery through the diseased cervix. Radiation therapy gives better survival figures than surgery. Cases are divided into three categories:

1. LESS THAN 28 WEEKS. The treatment should ignore the pregnancy and external radiation given to the entire pelvis. The foetus will abort spontaneously after about 3000 rads. A few days later radium may be inserted.

2. AFTER 28 WEEKS. Caesarian section followed by external radiotherapy, followed by radium insertion.

3. POST-PARTUM. External radiation followed by radium insertion.

Miscellaneous Tumours

Hodgkin's disease presenting as a lump in the neck can be treated by localised radiotherapy without risk. If a lymphoma presents as a lump in the groin, however, the dose to the foetus will obviously be significant. Most of the vital organs are formed by 12 weeks, but a dose of 25 rads can lead to blindness at 6 weeks gestation.

The problem is also difficult with carcinoma of the bladder and tumours lying in the pelvis. In these situations each case must be considered on its own merits. As a general rule, however, the pregnancy should be ignored if protection of the foetus compromises patient survival.

References

Dawson, W. B. *Growth impairment following radiography in childhood*, Clin. Radiol., 1968, **19**, 241.
Lowry, W. S. *Passive immunity against childhood cancer*, Lancet, 1974, **1**, 602.
Paterson, E. *Malignant tumours of childhood*, Clin. Radiol., 1958, **9**, 170.
Tefft, M. *Pediatric Tumour Refresher Course*, Radiol. Soc. N. Amer., 3 December, 1968, 410.

22

Benign Diseases

Radiotherapy is mostly concerned today with the treatment of malignant disease. Previously radiation was used to treat many other conditions such as syringomyelia, where it is of no value, tuberculosis where it is dangerous and peptic ulcer where, surprisingly, its value is not yet fully understood.

There are, however, a number of benign diseases where radiation therapy can be efficacious.

ANKYLOSING SPONDYLITIS

This hereditary condition of young men is a chronic inflammatory joint disease. It affects the sacro-iliac joints, the intervertebral and the costovertebral joints. As the disease progresses, the junction between the cortex and connective tissue is destroyed. Eventually repair takes place with ossification of the ligaments, and the joints become fused with bony ankylosis. The disease has a number of systemic manifestations.

Three clinical phases are recognized. The first phase lasts about 3 years, and the patient complains of lumbago and fleeting back pains. This is followed by an acute stage where the pain is severe and worse in the mornings. The condition is then said to 'burn itself out', leaving stiffness and deformity. Occasionally the disease may present in the elderly with stiffness and immobility without the painful inflammatory changes. This variant has been called senile hypertrophic ankylosing spondylopathy.

Radiographic Changes
1 Loss of spinal curvature.
2 Sacro-ilitis.
3 Calcification of ligaments.
4 'Squaring' of the vertebral bodies.
5 'Bamboo' spine.

Treatment
1 General measures.
2 Physiotherapy.

3 Drugs — aspirin and phenylbutazone have been used.
4 Radiation therapy.

Radiation gives dramatic pain relief within a few days, and most patients are enabled to return to work. The question of whether radiotherapy relieves stiffness is more difficult to assess since many cases seem to improve spontaneously.

Treatment is usually reserved for severe cases where other measures have failed. Some therapists recommend irradiating only the painful areas but others advise irradiation of the whole spine including the sacro-iliac joints. An inverted T-shaped field is usually recommended. Various dose schedules have been suggested ranging from 1500 rads in 3 weeks to 2000 rads in 2 weeks. Even smaller doses may be used, especially in the rare pre-menopausal female patient. Occasionally additional radiation may be given in case of intractable pain, but in no case should the total dose to the spine exceed 3000 rads.

Complications

Radiation therapy is known to cause late onset leukaemia in a small number of cases. The question is whether this slight risk is justified. Statisticians suggest that it is probably no greater than the risk of having an anaesthetic. Moreover, the hazard has to be balanced against the relief obtained and the alternative risks of drug therapy.

KELOIDS

There has been much discussion over the nature and treatment of true keloids and hypertrophic scars.

True keloids are more common in pigmented races. There is often a family history, and in some African villages almost every inhabitant has one or more keloids. They occur in response to trauma which may be quite trivial.

They are also found following surgery, usually where the incisions fail to parallel natural skin creases. True keloids are in fact benign collagen tissue neoplasms.

The recommended treatment today is an intra-lesional injection of hydrocortisone or triamcinolone. This will cure most cases. Where it fails, excision can be tried, followed by post-operative radiotherapy. Radiation should be given within 24 hours of the operation, before the fibroblasts divide. Superficial therapy is satisfactory, and the dose should not exceed 1500 rads in 10 days. Pre-operative radiation seems to be of no value.

The rare congenital keloid overlying the sternum should not be treated.

SKIN DISEASES

Generally speaking, most radiotherapists are reluctant to use radiation in the treatment of simple skin complaints. Certainly the cavernous haemangioma or 'strawberry' nevus should not be treated unless it is obstructing the airway or threatening vision. This lesion disappears spontaneously with time. The port-wine stain is not susceptible to any form of treatment and is best left alone.

Some dermatologists recommend small doses of Grenz rays for intractable skin diseases not responding to conventional measures. These conditions include:

1 Pustular psoriasis.
2 Chronic paronychia.
3 Pompholyx.
4 Neurodermatitis with lichenification.
5 Hyperhydrosis.

Small doses have been recommended, ranging from 400 rads in 4 days to 100 rads weekly for 5 weeks. These treatments may be repeated up to three times if necessary.

DISEASES OF THE EYE

Radiation has been recommended in the following simple eye conditions:

1 Corneal vascularization following corneal graft. Radiation is given by a strontium 90 beta shell applied directly to the eye. The dose given should be about 500 rads single. This can be repeated after a few days if necessary.
2 Intractable keratitis.
3 Corneal ulcers.

POST-HERPETIC NEURALGIA

This is a recognized complication of herpes zoster. A dose of 400 rads to the dorsal root ganglion may be given. This is thought to reduce gliosis and fibrosis and relieve pain. However, at least one large clinical trial recently failed to substantiate this claim.

RADIATION MENOPAUSE

Artificial induction of menopause may be necessary for menorrhagia in obese patients unsuitable for surgery. It may also be indicated for pre-menopausal patients with disseminated breast cancer and occasionally for patients with endometriosis that cannot be managed by other means.

The sterilizing dose is about 550 rads single to both ovaries or 1250 rads in 4 days. Younger women may require a somewhat higher dose. Field sizes average about 10 × 20 cm parallel opposed fields.

It should be noted that there is a 15-fold increase in the incidence of myocardial infarction in patients following surgical oophorectomy. This may also be true following radiation-induced menopause. Furthermore, a recent survey of cases treated by radiotherapy revealed several other late complications including malignant disease. In spite of these occasional sequelae, there may be no alternative to irradiation if debilitated anaemic patients are to be restored to health.

MISCELLANEOUS CONDITIONS

Small doses of radiation are occasionally helpful in the treatment of bursitis and shoulder tenosynovitis. A dose of 450 rads in three treatments is recommended. Radiation is of no value in the treatment of rheumatoid arthritis although there have been a few reports of its efficacy in osteoarthritis.

In Chicago and Boston two large series of patients with peptic ulcer were treated with doses up to 1500 rads in 10 days. This was found to reduce gastric acidity by about 50 per cent. However, the work has not been repeated elsewhere. There have also been reports that radiation therapy controls some cases of haematemesis not responding to surgery.

Radiation is of no value in the treatment of angina pectoris. Griseofulvin has replaced radiation therapy in the treatment of ringworm.

Painful bony involvement in Gaucher's disease may be relieved with small local palliative doses of radiation. Malignant exophthalmos and proptosis of the eye have been treated with radiation, but results are poor.

High-energy particles have been used to induce 'thalatomy' in Parkinson's disease. Pituitary ablation has been recommended in selected cases of diabetic retinopathy. There has also been a report of the use of radiotherapy in sub-acute sclerosing encephalitis.

Simple cavernous haemangioma of the liver may occasionally cause pressure symptoms. Small pedunculated lesions can be dealt with surgically. Larger lesions may require X-ray therapy; 3000 rads in 3 weeks is recommended. Care should be taken to avoid the kidney.

Small doses of radiation therapy have been used to treat pseudotumours in patients suffering from haemophilia.

Peyronie's disease is a distressing benign condition involving the penis. It seems resistant to all forms of therapy and, although pain can be relieved by radiation, few cures have been obtained.

IMMUNOSUPPRESSION

The problem of graft rejection following transplant surgery is still largely unsolved. The part that radiation should play is also unknown.

Two mechanisms may be involved in the rejection process. In the first, lymphocytes interact with graft antigens and invade and destroy homografts. In the second, immunoglobulins are laid down on graft capillaries. Platelets collect on these causing endothelial proliferation.

At the time of writing, the following methods have been used in an attempt to suppress the rejection process:

1. CYTOTOXIC DRUGS. Azathioprine ('Imuran') 5 mg/kg for 2 days orally. Thereafter 2·5 mg/kg.

2. STEROIDS. Prednisone 100 mg daily, dropping to 50 mg after 10 days.

3. ANTI-LYMPHOCYTIC SERUM. Prepared from horses injected with human lymphocytes.

4. EXTERNAL RADIATION. Whole body and splenic irradiation have been abandoned. Currently some clinicians recommend irradiation to the transplanted kidney following surgery. The suggested dose schedule is 450 rads in three divided doses of 150 rads on alternate days.

5. EXTRA-CORPOREAL IRRADIATION OF BLOOD (ECIB). This technique is still experimental. Heparinized blood is irradiated as it passes through a nylon tube. The technique employs the beta rays from a 24 curie strontium 90 source. A dose between 3000 and 18 000 rads/day is delivered continuously for several days. This produces a profound lymphopenia. The technique is thought to be effective in controlling early rejection phenomena but of little value for late rejection.

HYPERTHYROIDISM

This subject is adequately dealt with in most general medical textbooks. A few features of radiotherapeutic interest are discussed here.

Thyrotoxicosis may be treated by anti-thyroid drugs, surgery or ionizing radiation. Radioactive iodine provides a convenient means of delivering a high dose of radiation to the thyroid follicles with minimal damage to the surrounding tissues.

Radio-isotope therapy has been criticized because of the increased incidence of post-radiation hypothyroidism. However, this can be controlled with thyroid hormone replacement therapy.

The treatment dose of radioactive iodine may be calculated from tracer studies. The recommended therapeutic dose was originally about 10 000 rep. However, it is often difficult to measure the size of the gland and dosimetry errors of several hundred per cent may occur. Consequently some therapists now prescribe an empirical dose between 3 and 6 millicuries of radio-iodine.

This can be repeated if necessary. Massive ablation doses may also be given. Such treatment must automatically be followed by thyroid replacement therapy. This removes the necessity for long-term follow-up.

About one half of patients with thyrotoxicosis eventually revert spontaneously to euthyroidism. Presumably if radio-iodine is given to these patients, the gland will be permanently damaged, eventually producing inevitable hypothyroidism.

Radiobiologically, latent cell damage and death may not be seen until mitosis, long after irradiation. This correlates with the clinical findings of some physicians, who report that the development of post-radiation hypothyroidism is a continuing process, progressing at a rate of about 3 per cent per annum.

Several radioactive isotopes of iodine are now available. It has been suggested that the short-range particles from I^{125} may cause differential intracellular damage without cell death, giving a lower incidence of hypothyroidism. Initial experiments are disappointing however. A comparison of the different physical characteristics of the iodine isotopes was given in Chapter 2.

References

Dewing, S. B. *Radiotherapy of benign disease*, Charles C. Thomas, Springfield, Ill., 1965.

Fulton, J. S. *Ankylosing spondylitis*, Clin. Radiol., 1949, **1**, 67.

23

Recent Advances

HYPERBARIC OXYGEN

Most malignant tumours contain some anoxic cells. These cells are more radioresistant than oxygenated cells. It has been estimated that beyond 200 microns from the stromal blood supply the tumour is anoxic. This distance can be compared with a living cancer cell which is about 150 microns thick. The powerful influence of a small number of anoxic cells is illustrated by measuring the lethal dose required to kill 90 per cent of irradiated cells (TCD_{90}). Experiments show that the TCD_{90} for 1000 anoxic cells is greater than the TCD_{90} for 100 million aerobic cells.

It has been suggested that the radiosensitivity of anoxic tumours may be increased by making the patient breathe hyperbaric oxygen. At atmospheric pressure haemoglobin is normally over 95 per cent saturated. If the partial pressure is increased, however, oxygen dissolves in plasma.

Technique

Anaesthesia is usually omitted since no evidence of toxicity develops at a pressure of 3 atmospheres absolute. However anaesthesia is indicated for: (1) exposure, even at total rest, to oxygen pressures greater than 3 atmospheres; (2) apprehensive, anxious or claustrophobic patients; (3) patients with a cerebral tumour; (4) patients unable to lie still for long periods; (5) patients with a previous oxygen convulsion while conscious (oxygen convulsions are more common in the USA where, for legal reasons, patients are notified of this risk beforehand).

Since one-third of patients have trouble equalizing barometric pressure in the middle ear even if the pressure is elevated slowly and linearly, bilateral myringotomy is performed on most patients before treatment. Modified hypodermic needles are inserted through the tympanic membranes and remain in place during treatment.

The patient is at full pressure for 15 minutes before treatment starts. This permits saturation of the tumour tissue with oxygen. In anaesthetized patients, myringotomy is performed after induction of anaesthesia. This allows faster compression, and pressures of 4 atmospheres absolute can be attained in 6 to 7 minutes. The decompression rate is similar to that for conscious patients.

Dose

Simplified fractionation patterns had to be devised because of the length of each individual treatment under hyperbaric oxygen. Doses of the order of 3500 to 3750 rads in six treatments over 18 days have been used. In some cases higher doses have been employed, but if the irradiated region includes laryngeal cartilages, the maximum dose should not exceed the lower figure, otherwise cartilage necrosis develops. Additional complications include failure of tissue defects to heal, oxygen toxicity, otitic barotrauma and severe epithelial reactions.

Results

The early results of Dr Churchill-Davidson in London suggested that in 20 per cent of cases improvement is dramatic. Best results were obtained in head and neck cancer and advanced tumours of the uterine cervix. Response with brain tumours has been disappointing. The most noteworthy effects follow treatment of metastatic neck nodes which often resist standard radiotherapeutic techniques.

Controlled clinical trials are now going on in many centres. Conflicting reports have been given, but in at least one series of cases reported from Cardiff, the earlier encouraging results have been confirmed.

Hydrogen Peroxide Therapy

Attempts have been made to overcome tumour anoxia by injecting intra-arterial hydrogen peroxide. Results have not yet been fully assessed.

Hypoxic Therapy

An alternative method of overcoming tumour anoxia is to make the surrounding normal tissue hypoxic and then increase the radiation dose. This has been done in a case of osteogenic sarcoma by cooling the lower limb and applying a tourniquet. The dose can then be increased by a factor of 2·3. A total dose of 16 000 rads in 7 weeks has been suggested. Only a few sporadic cases have been treated in this way, and the technique has not been widely adopted.

NEUTRON THERAPY

Fast Neutrons

Fast neutrons are those with energies above 5 MeV. They may be produced by cyclotrons or other heavy particle accelerators. So far, there has been little clinical experience with fast neutron beams, but experiments suggest the following advantages over gamma ray therapy:

   1. Neutron beams consist of high LET radiation with an increased

RBE and a resultant low OER (see Chapter 3). Consequently the oxygen effect is less important with neutrons. However, the OER is not quite unity and the disadvantage of gamma radiation not fully eliminated. Recent work suggests a ratio of about 1·7 for neutrons compared with 2·8 for gamma radiation. Thus for the same degree of damage to normal aerobic tissues, fast neutrons will produce greater damage in anoxic tissues than gamma radiation.

2. With high LET radiation the shoulder 'N' disappears. As already indicated, this is probably because the passage of a single high LET particle is sufficient to kill the cell. With low LET radiation, multiple tracks arriving at different times allow inter-current repair of sub-lethal injury.

The disappearance of 'N' would suggest that fractionation of neutron therapy is less likely to help, but results are conflicting and further experiments will be necessary to resolve this question. Other factors also require clarification. Neutrons act by releasing heavy particles in tissue. These include deuterons, alpha particles and recoil nuclei. Hence energy is dissipated through a series of steps, and there is a wide range of LET and RBE. In biological work average values are usually taken. The biological effects are further complicated by the atomic structure of different tissues. For instance, fat has a large number of hydrogen atoms boosting dose absorption by 15 per cent. This could lead to subcutaneous necrosis. In spite of these potential drawbacks, neutrons offer interesting possibilities. A 14 MeV source would seem to provide the best beam for clinical purposes. Such a unit has now been designed and will be available shortly.

Slow Neutrons

Boron capture therapy using slow thermal neutrons has been used to treat brain tumours. If a slow neutron beam is directed at the brain, radioactivity may be induced in the boron atoms leading theoretically to sterilization of the tumour. Unfortunately boron uptake in brain tumours is disappointingly low. In addition, it is not yet possible to measure the radiation dose *in situ*.

HEAVY PARTICLE THERAPY

Heavy charged particles include deuterons, protons, pi-mesons and alpha particles. They have several advantages over gamma radiation (Table XII).

TABLE XII

Comparison with gamma radiation

	Neutrons	Protons	Pions	Heavy ions
Depth Dose	same	improved	improved	improved
OER	improved	same	improved	much improved

There is little scatter from charged particles and they produce virtually no skin damage. Neutrons on the other hand have a similar depth dose distribution to megavoltage X-rays.

Protons have a characteristic Bragg-peak depth dose curve (Figure 28). The position of this peak depends on the proton beam energy and can be varied to fit the particular clinical situation. The integral dose is lower, enabling the therapist to deliver a highly effective dose to the tumour volume with minimal damage to surrounding normal tissue. The technique has not yet been fully exploited.

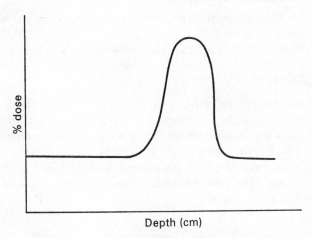

Figure 28   Proton Bragg-peak dosage curve

Negative pi-mesons lose their energy by exploding as alpha particles at the ends of their tracks. They are largely insensitive to oxygen and there is no recovery from sub-lethal injury. The short range fragments produced in the tumour have a relatively high LET. 190 MeV deuterons, 340 MeV protons and 910 MeV alpha particles have all been used to treat various conditions ranging from brain tumours to Parkinson's disease. Diabetic retinopathy, acromegaly and metastatic breast tumours have been treated by radiation hypophysectomy using massive single exposures of up to 8000 rads.

Unfortunately these machines are costly and are not readily available for clinical work. Nevertheless one-third of all patients with cancer still die from local disease, and it is possible that heavy particle therapy may be substantially better than gamma radiation for these patients.

ELECTRONS

Low-energy electrons are emitted from certain radioactive isotopes such as yttrium 90. Medium energies (2–10 MeV) may be obtained from the linear accelerator. Higher energies can be generated in a betatron.

G

Electron beams have the following advantages over gamma ray therapy:

1 Low integral dose.
2 The beam terminates abruptly with no exit dose.
3 Low skin dose, homogeneous absorption and good penetration.
4 Flat isodose curves allow easy dosimetry.
5 The penetration is largely independent of SSD.
6 The penetration is proportional to beam energy affording easy control.

The disadvantages of electron therapy are:

1 The clinical response has not been fully worked out and more experience is needed.
2 There is a variable RBE and the biological effects are largely unknown.
3 Scatter leads to uneven dose distribution and can make protection difficult.

Electron therapy has been suggested for tumours of the head and neck including the parotid gland, antrum, tonsil and brain. Other sites where a sharp cut-off is required include the female urethra and the external auditory meatus and neck nodes overlying the spinal cord.

An electron beam of 3 MeV is a convenient method for treating mycosis fungoides, a superficial skin condition. Electron beams are also of value in treating the perineal region.

AFTERLOADING

Afterloading consists of inserting inactive intracavitary applicators or interstitial needles into the tumour. When a satisfactory geometrical arrangement has been obtained, the hollow applicators are loaded with the radioactive sources. The advantages of afterloading are:

1 Reduced radiation hazard to staff.
2 It allows the operator more time to ensure meticulous technique.
3 The total treatment time can be considerably reduced by using stronger radiation sources.

The disadvantages of afterloading are:

1 Improper loading and 'sticking' occasionally lead to excessive exposure.
2 The radiobiological effects of the different radioactive isotopes are not fully known.

Interstitial Implants

1. REMOVABLE IMPLANTS. Hollow steel needles are inserted in the lesion and held in place by plastic stabilisers (Figure 29). When the geometrical

arrangement is satisfactory, a suitable radioactive isotope is introduced into the shafts of the needles. Iridium 192 seeds, spaced 1 cm apart in nylon ribbons, have been used. The nylon ribbons can be cut to the required size in the operating room. Removable implants can be used in any situation where radium might have been used (eg, tongue). The time of the insertion can be altered according to the distribution of the needles and the dose required.

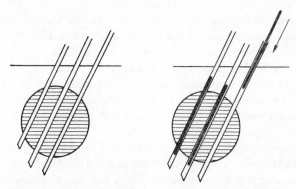

Figure 29   Afterloading of hollow-shafted needles

2. PERMANENT IMPLANTS. 15 cm hollow needles are inserted into the tumour. Since they are not radioactive they can be guided into position by carefully palpating below the lesion with the finger tips. The required seed distribution is then calculated. A special introducer with a depth gauge is attached to each needle in turn. The plunger is pressed and the needle withdrawn the required distance after each shot, leaving a seed behind. Radioactive gold seeds, Au^{198}, are convenient. The method is simple and quick and there is often no need to admit the patient to the hospital.

The technique is indicated in any situation where radon seeds might have been used, for instance a small lesion on the floor of the mouth.

Intracavitary Therapy
Special hollow applicators are inserted into the uterine canal and lateral fornices. Bladder and rectal dose readings can be taken with calibrated microsources in place. Verification X-ray films are made of the dummy sources. Depending on the radiographic appearance of the system, any necessary changes in loading can still be made. If the position is satisfactory the active sources are inserted later on the ward in less than 30 seconds. The technique is particularly suitable for the Fletcher-Suit applicators after-loaded with caesium, and is used increasingly.

The Cathetron
This remote-control device has been used in the treatment of carcinoma of the endometrium.

The patient is sedated or anaesthetized and placed in the lithotomy position. Specially-manufactured 'Manchester' catheters are inserted into the uterine canal and vaginal fornices. These are held rigidly and connected by nylon tubes to remote cobalt 60 sources (5 curie tubes and 2·5 curie ovoids). When gauze packing is used the uterus may slip off the fixed uterine catheter. Thus a special rectal retractor is required for the posterior wall of the vagina.

A monitor scintillation counter is placed in the rectum and a small tracer dose of Cobalt 60 injected through the nylon tubes. Dose rate measurements are made at 1 cm intervals along the rectum and the insertion arranged so that the dose is adjusted to 60 per cent of that at Point A.

The scintillation counter is then removed and replaced by a high-intensity cadmium sulphide rectal probe. Check X-rays are taken. The room is then vacated and the high-intensity cobalt sources injected into the catheters.

The dose rate to the vaginal epithelium is about 450 rads/min with 180 rads/min to Point A and 55 rads/min to Point B. Total treatment time varies between 20 minutes and half an hour. Provisional treatments aim at delivering 5000 rads to Point A in 10 fractions over 24 hours. Since the clinical results have not yet been fully assessed, the technique has mainly been used pre-operatively.

More recently the technique has been used in carcinoma of the cervix. Combined intracavitary and external treatments give doses of up to 12 000 rads to the cervix and 4000 rads to the pelvic wall. This is achieved over 3 weeks by 4 intracavitary applications and 12 external treatments. Preliminary results seem to be as good as conventional methods of treatment. An added advantage of the cathetron is that patients do not need to be confined to bed.

References

Afterloading in Radiotherapy, Conference Proceedings, 1971, U.S. Dept. H.E.W., #72–8024.

Duncan, W. *Neutron Therapy*, Brit. J. Hosp. Med., 1969, **2**, 1486.

Henk, J. M., *et al. Hyperbaric oxygen in radiotherapy*, Clin. Radiol., 1970, **21**, 223.

Joslin, C. A., O'Connell, D., and Howard N. *Treatment of uterine carcinoma using the Cathetron*, Brit. J. Radiol., 1967, **40**, 882.

Suit, H. D., Moore, E. B., Fletcher, G. H., and Worsnop, R. *An Afterloading System for cervical cancer*, Radiology, 1963, **81**, 126.

24

Cancer Chemotherapy

The division of radiotherapy and cancer chemotherapy into two separate subjects is partly artificial. Radiotherapy is a form of chemotherapy. As already explained, discrete packets of radiation energy are delivered into living cells where the quanta are transformed into ion-pairs creating highly reactive chemical radicals. It is not surprising, therefore, that many cytotoxic drugs act in a similar way to radiation and indeed the alkylating agents have been called radiomimetic drugs.

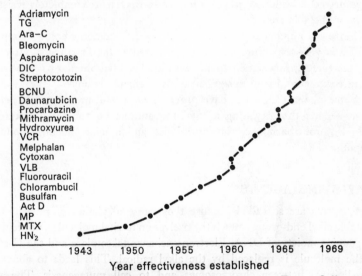

Figure 30   **Clinically effective anti-tumour agents. Rate of discovery**

Yet cytotoxic therapy has come a long way from the discovery of alkylating agents. Just how far is illustrated by the rate at which clinically effective drugs are being discovered (Figure 30) (Frei). On this graph, 23 useful drugs are listed in ascending order. On the horizontal axis, the year in which the efficacy of the drug was established is presented, starting with nitrogen mustard in 1943. During the 1950s the number of agents increased gradually and during the 1960s rapidly.

Long-term remissions and occasional chemotherapeutic cures are now being obtained in several forms of cancer (Table XIII). It is of interest that these are mostly diseases of relatively young people. Unfortunately they are also among the rarer types of malignancy. On the other hand the list represents some of the most highly malignant forms of cancer.

TABLE XIII

Diseases highly responsive to chemotherapy (Zubrod)

Burkitt's lymphoma	Embryonal testicular cancer
Choriocarcinoma	Wilm's tumour
Acute lymphocytic leukaemia	Ewing's sarcoma
Hodgkin's disease	Rhabdomyosarcoma
Lymphosarcoma	Retinoblastoma
Mycosis fungoides	

Results in solid tumours have been less impressive. In this group of diseases, the chief value of cytotoxic therapy lies in restoring the patient to temporary good health. A proportion of cases treated are completely resistant for no predictable reason.

Since the number of cancer cases cured by chemotherapy is relatively small, it is vital that drugs should not be used as the first line of attack in early disease. Already some patients with localized lymphomas have forfeited a chance of a cure due to misguided trials of chemotherapy.

Some of the drugs that have proved most useful are discussed below. These include the alkylating agents, the antimetabolites, the vinca rosea alkaloids, procarbazine, certain antibiotics and a miscellaneous group of compounds.

ALKYLATING AGENTS

These agents are so called because they cause alkylation of nucleic acid. Unstable alkyl end-groups attach themselves on to vital molecules, particularly the guanine moiety of DNA. Electron exchange takes place and the H-atom on the molecule is replaced by the alkyl radical. This leads to abnormal cross-linkages between chromosomes and to cell mutagenesis. The new alkylating agents are lipid-soluble and distribute freely. This enables them to reach malignant cells not undergoing division at the time of treatment.

Most of the alkylating agents in clinical use are modifications of the basic mustard structure:

$$R - N = (Cl - CH_2 - CH_2)_2.$$

By altering the chain length, various drugs have been derived from the parent compound.

Mechlorethamine (Nitrogen Mustard)

This was the first chemotherapeutic agent to be used in cancer. The drug is still useful in Hodgkin's disease and many other conditions. Solutions of mustine hydrochloride must be freshly prepared before use. Care should be taken in handling this drug since it is highly vesicant. It must be given intravenously since extravasation causes local tissue necrosis. Nitrogen mustard is highly toxic and acts rapidly. The recommended dose is about 0·2–0·4 mg/kg in divided doses.

Cyclophosphamide (Endoxana)

This drug has a low hydrolysis but liver enzymes split off the phosphoramide derivative in the body releasing dichloroethylamine. Cyclophosphamide is one of the most widely used cytotoxic drugs. It has the broadest spectrum of all the alkylating agents. The drug is well tolerated orally in doses of up to 200 mg daily. Higher doses, up to 15 mg/kg weekly may be given parenterally. Side-effects include nausea, bone marrow depression, haematuria and alopecia. These are discussed in more detail later. There is evidence that phenobarbital given beforehand can mobilize liver enzymes for quicker activation of the drug.

Phenylalanine Mustard (PAM, Melphalan, Alkeran)

This compound is derived from the amino acid phenylalanine. It was synthesized in the hope that it would be specific for malignant melanoma. Unfortunately this hope was not realized but the drug has been used extensively in the treatment of multiple myeloma. It is well absorbed by the oral route. Up to 10 mg daily can usually be tolerated for short periods. The recommended intravenous dosage is about 1 mg/kg.

Chlorambucil (Leukeran)

This drug has a longer biological half-life in serum than mustard. It has been used extensively in chronic lymphatic leukaemia, carcinoma of the ovary and carcinoma of the breast. The compound is less toxic than the other alkylating agents but this may be partly due to the dose levels used, since it is also less effective. The recommended oral dosage is 6–15 mg daily.

Ethoglicid (Epodyl)

This drug is known to cross the blood-brain barrier and is used in the treatment of cerebral tumours. It may be given intravenously or arterially.

Ethyleneimines

These compounds were derived from the textile industry where they are used as textile 'cross-linkers'. The best known are Tretamine (TEM) and Thiotepa. They resemble chemically the active substance produced when nitrogen mustards are dissolved in water.

TRETAMINE (TEM). This compound can be given orally. It is less toxic to the liver than nitrogen mustard. However it is a severe bone marrow depressant. The drug has been used to supplement radiation therapy in the treatment of retinoblastoma. Variable results have been reported.

THIOTEPA. The drug has been widely used but appears to have no special advantage over the alkylating agents.

Di-Methane Sulphonates

The di-methane sulphonates are chemically unrelated to the mustards. Their precise mode of action is unknown but it does not involve interstrand cross-linkage with DNA. Most of the oncolytic effect may be due to reactions with thiol groups in proteins.

BUSULPHAN (MYELERAN). This is the best-known compound of the series. Busulphan resembles radiation more closely than the other alkylating agents. In this sense, it is close to being a true radiomimetic drug. It is the drug of choice in myeloid leukaemia and is well absorbed orally. A dose of 5 mg daily may be given for up to 3 months or longer. Long-term follow-up has shown a number of disturbing side-effects including pulmonary fibrosis, pigmentation, an Addisonian-like wasting and amenorrhoea.

ANTIMETABOLITES

These drugs block the synthesis of nucleic acid, preventing its incorporation into nucleoprotein. They act by competitive inhibition. That is, they are sufficiently like a normal metabolite to combine with the same enzymes, but sufficiently different to prevent the usual metabolic reaction. The concept is analagous to the mode of action of sulphonamides. Thus antimetabolites are 'carcinostatic' rather than 'carcinocidal'. For this reason, they are indicated when malignant cells are multiplying rapidly, as in acute leukaemia (cell doubling time is 3 days). The average doubling time in most malignant tumours is about four months.

The folic acid inhibitors were among the first antimetabolites discovered. Subsequently antagonists of pyrimidine and other base analogues were described.

Methotrexate

This drug is used in the treatment of a number of conditions including acute leukaemia, choriocarcinoma, head and neck tumours and breast carcinoma. Toxic effects appear when the dose exceeds 10 mg/day. These are first seen in the rapidly dividing cells of the mouth where the patient develops stomatitis, gingivitis and pharyngitis. Side-effects are numerous and include alopecia, gastrointestinal upset, acute liver atrophy, hypogammaglobulinaemia and serositis. Liver damage may be detected up to 6 months after cessation of therapy. The effects of methotrexate can be reversed by giving the antidote, citrovorum factor (see later).

Recent work has shown that vincristine given 30 minutes before methotrexate improves cell membrane transport and uptake.

6-mercaptopurine

6-MP is an analogue of the purine base adenine. The drug is well absorbed orally. It is used extensively in the treatment of acute leukaemia. Side-effects are less severe than with methotrexate but include diarrhoea and sprue-like symptoms. Reports suggest that a higher proportion of children than adults respond favourably.

Azathiopurine (Imuran)

This drug is broken down *in vivo* into 6-MP and is thought to be less toxic. It is mainly metabolized to 6-thiouric acid. Azathiopurine is mostly used as an immunosuppressive agent following transplant surgery but like the other antimetabolites it acts on all dividing cells.

5-fluorouracil

5-FU is a fluorinated pyrimidine. It blocks methylation of deoxyuridilic acid and interferes with DNA synthesis. The drug is mostly used in the treatment of inoperable gastro-intestinal malignancies. Variable results are reported. 5-FU is extremely toxic. Originally the recommended dose was 15 mg/kg daily for 4 days in an intravenous infusion containing glucose. However it has been suggested that a small weekly dose of 1–2 mg/kg is equally effective and less toxic. Thereafter the dose may be reduced to 7·5 mg/kg on alternate days until the 12th day, unless toxicity supervenes.

Other antimetabolites that have been tried include 6-azauracil and cytarabine. They have no special advantage over those already mentioned.

VINCA ROSEA ALKALOIDS

Vincristine and vinblastine are natural alkaloids extracted from the periwinkle plant, Vinca Rosea. Both molecules are large and have a similar structure and mechanism of action. Vinblastine interferes with the metabolic pathway leading from glutamic acid to the citric acid cycle and urea. Both drugs block cellular growth at metaphase. There is no cross-resistance with other oncolytic agents. Vinblastine has often produced fresh remissions in Hodgkin's disease when other drugs have failed. The recommended dose is 10 mg intravenously weekly. Side-effects are uncommon.

Vincristine is indicated in the treatment of several diseases including acute leukaemia in childhood. An important side-effect is peripheral neuropathy. It has much less marrow toxicity than vinblastine.

PROCARBAZINE

This drug is related to the anti-depressive group of drugs known as mono-amine oxidase inhibitors. Its anti-tumour effect is probably due to the formation of hydrogen peroxide and hydroxyl radicals within the cells. This leads to denaturation of DNA. There is no cross-resistance with other oncolytic agents. Procarbazine has been used in Hodgkin's disease to obtain additional remissions when other drugs have failed. It is thought to be especially valuable when the bone marrow is severely depressed.

ASPARAGINASE

Asparagine is essential for cellular metabolism. Normal cells manufacture it for themselves from asparitic acid and glutamine, but cancer cells are unable to do so and rely on exogenous supplies. Asparaginase destroys exogenous asparagine. Attempts have been made to use this enzyme as a therapeutic tool to destroy malignant cells. The substance is expensive and its clinical application is at present limited to studies on leukaemia patients. It is now known that this dependence of tumour cells on a normal metabolite is not an isolated abnormality, and we may yet be able to exploit other examples of the phenomenon.

ANTIBIOTICS

A number of compounds of fungal origin were found to be oncolytic. Their cytotoxic properties precluded their use in the treatment of infectious disease.

Actinomycin D

This drug inhibits RNA synthesis by binding to the site of the DNA template, where RNA polymerase functions. It also inhibits DNA synthesis. Actinomycin D is recommended in the treatment of Wilm's tumour. A dose of 15 mg/kg daily intravenously for 5 days is suggested. A second course of treatment may be given after an interval of 2 weeks. Thereafter various dose schedules have been described (see later). A variety of abnormalities may follow its use. These effects may not become apparent until 3 days after treatment has stopped. The compound has also been recommended in a number of other conditions such as rhabdomyosarcoma, choriocarcinoma, testicular tumours and soft tissue sarcomas.

Bleomycin

This drug was discovered in Japan. It consists of a group of glycopeptides which are a mixture of related antibiotics. Bleomycin exerts its maximum effect during mitosis. Encouraging results have been obtained in epidermoid cancer of the head and neck, lung and oesophagus. It has also been used in Hodgkin's disease. The recommended dose is 10 mg/M^2/day intravenously.

The most disturbing side-effect is pulmonary fibrosis which develops in 5 to 10 per cent of cases.

Adriamycin
This tetracycline derivative is said to be effective in carcinoma of the bladder, breast and the lymphomas. It belongs to the anthracycline group of antibiotics and is related to daunorubicin. This latter drug is useful in acute myeloid leukaemia.

Actinomycin C
This compound has also been used as an immunosuppressive agent.

Mitomycin C
This drug can be considered metabolically as a derivative of ethyleneimine and urethane.

Mithramycin
This antibiotic is very toxic. Side-effects include hypocalcaemia. It is the drug of choice in embryonal cell carcinoma of the testis but is of little or no value in other testicular tumours.

MISCELLANEOUS COMPOUNDS
Thousands of compounds have been screened for cytotoxic activity. It would be futile to attempt an exhaustive list. Some of those that have been used include:

Arabinosyl Cystosine (Ara C)
This drug acts specifically during mitosis. As such it is cell-cycle specific. Ara C inhibits DNA formation by blocking DNA polymerase. The drug is inactive orally and must be given intravenously. It is useful in several forms of cancer including meningeal leukaemia. The compound is also schedule-dependent (see later).

Urethane (Ethyl Carbamate)
This sedative is metabolized to the active compound N-hydroxyurethane. It was originally used in multiple myeloma but is probably valueless.

Vitamin B12
Occasional dramatic remissions were originally reported in neuroblastoma but these were probably spurious.

Pyrimethamine (Daraprim)
This anti-malarial drug is sometimes used in polycythaemia.

Colchicine

This drug is known to induce mitotic delay. It has occasionally been used in cancer therapy.

Mitoclomine

This compound may be of value in malignant melanoma.

O, P'DDD (Mitotane)

This drug is specific for some cases of adrenal carcinoma.

Imidazole Carboxamide (DTIC)

Limited success has been obtained in malignant melanoma.

NEW DRUGS

Burchenal and Carter have divided new drugs into four groups:

1. PROVEN CLINICAL VALUE. Some of these compounds were discussed above. They include adriamycin, DTIC, bleomycin and asparaginase. Also included in this group are the nitrosoureas BCNU and CCNU. These latter drugs have proved useful in advanced breast cancer. BCNU is also known to cross the blood-brain barrier.

2. SUGGESTIVE CLINICAL VALUE. These include Streptozotocin, N-demethylepipodophyllotoxin thenylidine glucoside (VM-26), 5-azacytidine, hydroxyurea, guanazole and 5-hydroxypicolinaldehyde thisemicarbazone (5-HP).

3. AGENTS UNDER CLINICAL TRIAL. These consist of methyl-CCNU, ICRF 159, Iphosfamide, platinum diamminodichloride, and N-demethyl-epipodophyllotoxin ethylidine glucoside (VP-16).

4. PROMISING DRUGS BUT AS YET UNTESTED IN HUMANS. This group includes palmo ara-C; cyclo-cytidine; 2,2'-anhydro-1-(B-D-arabinosyl) 5-fluorocytosine.

INDICATIONS FOR CHEMOTHERAPY

There are now several types of cancer where chemotherapy is the treatment of choice. These include Burkitt's lymphoma, choriocarcinoma and acute lymphoblastic leukaemia.

In a number of other diseases, chemotherapy is indicated in conjunction with surgery or radiation therapy. Such conditions include Wilm's tumour and Ewing's sarcoma. A problem arises where the patient has early disease and may do well with surgery or radiation alone. Although chemotherapy can extend life, one is often not sure which patients need drugs and which do not. For instance, is it better to treat all cases of Wilm's tumour with potent chemotherapeutic agents and incur the risks of inducing unknown late effects in those that did not require chemotherapy in the first place? Or is it better to withhold therapy until the need is manifest, and then mount a massive therapeutic onslaught incorporating chemotherapy, possible repetitive surgery and radiation therapy with their undoubted attendant risks? The former course penalizes the child who would have done well without chemotherapy; the latter jeopardizes the patient who might have been better treated more simply with chemotherapy initially (D'Angio).

The commonest indication for chemotherapy is the patient who develops generalized metastatic carcinoma. Occasionally treatment may be withheld until such a patient develops symptoms. This concept is based on the aphorism, 'palliative therapy should only be given to those with symptoms to palliate'. However there is now evidence that in some types of cancer, it is better to initiate chemotherapy once metastatic disease has been diagnosed, even if the patient is asymptomatic.

In those patients who are treated one must remember that prolongation of life should be accompanied by an improvement in the quality of life. It is not enough to lengthen survival if the patient is perpetually sick from iatrogenic side-effects.

It is appropriate here to mention the controversial use of cytotoxic drugs in the treatment of non-malignant disease. These compounds have been used occasionally in the auto-immune conditions in an attempt to produce immunosuppression. In view of the serious side-effects of cytotoxic drugs the indications for treatment must await full clinical trials. Meanwhile there is a suggestion that cytotoxic therapy may be of value in certain cases of the nephrotic syndrome and possibly also severe rheumatoid arthritis. The indiscriminate use of cytotoxic drugs in such conditions as psoriasis, however, is to be condemned.

Dose

Many of the claims made for different cytotoxic drugs are probably due to different dose levels used, rather than inherent properties of the drugs themselves. In contrasting different drugs it is therefore important to compare optimal rather than equal doses. The recommended dose is usually the maximum the patient will tolerate. This is often limited by the toxic effects of the drug, such as depression of the bone marrow. As a rule of thumb, many clinicians accept a peripheral white cell count of 2000 as a borderline lower limit.

In a few diseases, judging the correct dose can be difficult. For instance in choriocarcinoma, cytotoxic drugs probably act differentially by eradicating rapidly dividing malignant cells without damaging normal immunocompetent cells.

The concept of schedule dependence is discussed later.

Length of Treatment

A second question to be considered is how long should chemotherapy be continued after a remission has been obtained. Generally speaking when cancer is clinically evident, there are 1×10^{12} tumour cells in the body. If treatment reduces the number to 1×10^9 cells, the tumour is usually too small to detect. So although there is an apparent complete remission, one billion tumour cells remain. How long and how intensively should therapy be continued after this point? In acute lymphocytic leukaemia, therapy is subsequently recommended for up to 2 years. Is this too much treatment or too little? The solution to the problem is suggested by choriocarcinoma. This neoplasm produces a chemical hormone, gonadotrophin. Quantitative assays make it possible to titrate treatment in choriocarcinoma until the last trace of gonadotrophin disappears from the urine. This would seem to be an ideal way of monitoring all chemotherapy, and there is an intensive search for similar products in other diseases. The search is not confined to chemical compounds and immunological factors such as tumour antigens are also being sought (Zubrod).

Choice of Compound

In some diseases certain compounds are recommended as the drugs of choice. Examples include actinomycin D for Wilm's tumour, cyclophosphamide for Burkitt's lymphoma and O, P′DDD for adrenal carcinoma. However in most forms of cancer the ideal drug has yet to be found. Often the choice of compound is a matter of personal taste and experience on the part of the physician.

Combination Chemotherapy

If a patient undergoing chemotherapy with one drug relapses, another drug may be tried. Cross-resistance between drugs of the same group can occur, but cyclical therapy with drugs of a different group may produce fresh remissions. If four drugs are known to be useful individually in a certain disease, one would anticipate a higher remission rate lasting a longer time when the same four drugs are given concurrently. Thus in comparing combination therapy with sequential therapy, it is important to show that such effects are synergistic and not simply additive. This subject is being investigated and is discussed later in the chapter. Meanwhile synergism has been demonstrated in the treatment of several diseases, including acute lymphoblastic leukaemia, Hodgkin's disease and breast carcinoma. Two examples are given below.

The Cooper Drug Programme for breast cancer involves giving the following drugs simultaneously:

Vincristine: 0·015 mg/kg/week intravenously.
Methotrexate: 15–50 mg/kg/week intravenously.

5-fluorouracil: 7·5 mg/kg/week intravenously.
Cytoxin: 50–150 mg/day orally.
Prednisone: 20–40 mg/day orally.

The MOPP Programme for Hodgkin's disease:

Mustard: 6 mg/M²/week intravenously.
Vincristine: 1·4 mg/M²/week intravenously.
Procarbazine: 100 mg/M²/day orally.
Prednisone: 40 mg/M²/day orally.

Citrovorum Rescue Programme

As already mentioned, the toxic effects of methotrexate can be reversed by giving citrovorum factor. A technique has been devised whereby massive supralethal doses of over 1 g of methotrexate can be given to patients with advanced disease. Citrovorum factor is then given up to 6 hours after the infusion of methotrexate. In this way the toxic side-effects can be decreased considerably. The technique has been used with encouraging results in patients with lung cancer and metastatic osteogenic sarcoma. The exact dose schedules and time intervals are currently under investigation.

REGIONAL CHEMOTHERAPY

Perfusion

Cancer chemotherapy may be limited to one region of the body by arterial perfusion. For this purpose an extra-corporeal circulation is required (Figure 31).

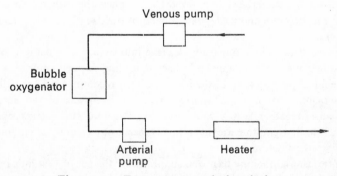

Figure 31   Extra-corporeal circulation

The patient is heparinized and the circuit primed with an autotransfusion of 700 cc of the patient's own blood. Arterial perfusion is usually given in sessions lasting about 1 hour. When the time exceeds this, there is often a 'leak' through anastomosing vessels to the systemic circulation. The role of oxygen is unsettled in perfusion, but it may be worth warming the limb while keeping the rest of the patient under hypothermia. The patient is usually anaesthetized for the procedure. Fluorescein dye and ultra-violet photography may be used beforehand to outline the treatment area.

Alkylating agents are recommended in up to eight times the normal dosage. Antimetabolites are of little value since they take a much longer time to act. The bone marrow can be aspirated before treatment. It may then be stored and autotransplanted later.

Regional perfusion can be performed in the limbs, head and neck, brain, lungs, liver and breast. The pelvis can also be isolated for treatment by preventing venous return with saline pressure in the peridural space.

Following treatment, the region may be flushed out with plasma. Local-tissue tolerance may develop with long-acting drugs such as cyclophosphamide.

Complications include leg oedema, wound infection, haematoma and general cytotoxic side-effects. Surprisingly thrombosis is rare.

Infusion

With this technique, continuous or intermittent arterial injection of drugs is possible for periods of up to several months. Methotrexate has been used extensively. Folinic acid may be given simultaneously to block the systemic effects. Up to 1000 ml of 5 per cent dextrose are infused under pressures of 60 mm Hg or higher. Fluorouracil and dactinomycin have also been used for infusion. Currently 5-FU is being used to control gastro-intestinal and liver metastases in some cases.

The most common regions treated are the lower limbs through the external iliac artery, the head and neck via the carotid artery and the liver through the hepatic artery. It is important to place the catheter far enough back in the artery to allow adequate mixing of the drug before it reaches the target area.

Side-effects include mucositis, leakage into tissues with painless blistering and oedema of the tongue and pharynx leading to pneumonia.

Regional perfusion and infusion have been recommended for palliation of malignant melanoma, metastatic squamous carcinoma of the head and neck, and fungating malodorous growths. Patients with intractable pain often do well. Symptomatic liver metastases from colonic carcinoma also receive good palliation.

Intra-arterial therapy has been simplified by the use of Watkin's infusor, a small clockwork infusion pump, which can be attached to the patient's clothing allowing full mobility during treatment.

SIDE-EFFECTS

Cytotoxic drugs are not specific for cancer cells. They also damage normal cells and give rise to numerous unwanted effects. In addition they may cause the usual allergic reactions obtained with any drug. Again these compounds are mutagenic and teratogenic and are dangerous in pregnancy. Their effects may be cumulative and it is probably unwise to use them in any woman of child-bearing age unless absolutely necessary. Not surprisingly, many of the unwanted effects of the so-called radiomimetic drugs resemble radiation damage.

Rapidly dividing cells are the first to be affected by radiation and cytotoxic drugs. These include epithelial cells lining the gastro-intestinal tract and bone marrow cells. Thus after relatively low doses patients may complain of anorexia, nausea and occasionally vomiting. Shortly after this, they develop leukopenia, associated with an increased tendency to mycotic and other infections. This may be accompanied by thrombocytopenia and episodes of bleeding. With slightly larger doses of radiation or drugs, temporary alopecia occurs and ovarian and testicular function is impaired.

Higher doses of radiation produce a number of pathological changes including pneumonitis, nephritis, hepatitis, myelitis and a protein-losing gastroenteropathy. These effects have all been described following long-term cytotoxic therapy. Some of these such as pulmonary fibrosis with busulphan, were previously thought to be specific, but this side-effect has now been seen with cyclophosphamide. By the same token, the syndrome 'transplant lung', previously considered an immunological cross-reaction, may be a simple side-effect of azathioprine, analogous to radiation pneumonitis.

Both radiation and cytotoxic drugs suppress the body's immune response. Recently a case of fatal systemic measles was reported in a child taking cyclophosphamide for the nephrotic syndrome.

At low dose levels, sub-lethal radiation damage may be reversible but higher doses produce permanent damage. These effects are cumulative. Hence it is not surprising to find that cytotoxic drugs occasionally potentiate the action of radiation and there have been reports of patients on cytotoxic drugs developing local tissue necrosis in previously irradiated areas.

Two further points are worth recalling: chronic exposure to low doses of radiation over many years can cause cancer; it can also cause long-term genetic damage. It is likely that many of the cytotoxic drugs will be equally hazardous. It has already been noted that nitrogen mustard predisposes to lung cancer. Again, patients on 'immunosuppressive' drugs have an increased risk of malignancy.

Nevertheless the term radiomimetic must not be applied indiscriminately. For instance, although antimetabolites may produce similar side-effects to the alkylating agents, they act earlier on rapidly dividing cells and the timing of onset of symptoms may be different. Thus methotrexate produces severe mouth reactions but leaves nerve and muscle cells largely unaffected. Moreover as already noted, in some cases the effect can be reversed by giving an antidote such as citrovorum factor.

Additional side-effects, not connected with those already discussed, have been described with some of the new drugs. Examples include pro-carbazine, a derivative of methyl hydrazine, which may potentiate barbiturates, phenothiazines and alcohol. Again, sparsomycin may cause a toxic retinopathy apparently due to degeneration of retinal pigment epithelium. It is also difficult to explain the relatively high incidence of neuromuscular disturb-ances associated with vincristine.

Finally there have been reports of the ingenious use of cyclophosphamide for sheep shearing. Although the quality of the wool may be unchanged, the mutton must surely be unfit for human consumption!

STEROIDS

Cortisone and its analogues have been used extensively in the treatment of malignant disease. They are specifically indicated in chronic lymphatic leukaemia where steroids are known to be lympholytic. Steroids are also used in haemolytic anaemia secondary to neoplastic disease and in hypercalcaemia. Cerebral oedema is an indication for steroid therapy. Good remissions have sometimes been obtained in other conditions such as Hodgkin's disease, multiple myeloma and metastatic breast cancer.

HORMONES

Hormonal therapy has been discussed under the various tumour headings. The main indications are in:

Breast cancer.
Endometrial cancer.
Prostatic cancer.
Thyroid cancer.

Hormone therapy has also been used in several other malignancies, notably hypernephroma, but results are not particularly encouraging.

IMMUNOTHERAPY

A full discussion of immunotherapy is beyond the scope of this book. For one thing, the subject is moving so rapidly that anything written today may be out of date tomorrow. Several general remarks are pertinent however.

The concept of immunotherapy presupposes that tumour cells are 'foreign' to the body and can theoretically be immunologically rejected. This may not be true for all forms of cancer.

It has been noted that enthusiasm for immunotherapy has gone through three phases in this century: optimism, pessimism and now realism. We are probably far enough into the modern phase of immunotherapy to make a cautious prediction, namely that immunotherapy will play an important part in the management of some cancer patients but will be no panacea. It seems likely that its role will be analogous to hormonal therapy and will probably be crucial in such tumours as neuroblastoma, malignant melanoma and possibly also lymphomas.

Potential methods of tumour immunotherapy have been sub-divided into six main groups. These are shown in Table XIV (after Currie).

TABLE XIV

Potential methods of immunotherapy

	Specific	Non-specific
Passive	Xenogeneic or allogeneic antisera.	Non-specific serum factors. Properdin, gamma globulin, etc.
Adoptive	Xenogeneic or allogeneic sensitized lymphoid cells or extracts.	Normal lymphoid cells — allogeneic or xenogeneic. Anti-tumour effect of GVH disease.
Active	Tumour cell vaccines: Living cells Attenuated cells Tumour antigens Foetal antigens	General stimulants of the immune response. BCG, C. parvum, Freund's adjuvant, etc.

FUTURE DEVELOPMENTS

One aim of cancer chemotherapy is to develop a drug that will selectively concentrate in malignant cells. Yet until we know more about the differences between normal and malignant cells this will be difficult.

Nevertheless cancer chemotherapy is moving away from the relatively sterile pursuit of endlessly testing different drugs. Frei has outlined the direction of future developments. These include more rational empiricism, better prediction systems in experimental animals, developments in cyto-kinetics, studies of chemical structure and advances in molecular biology.

1. Prediction Systems

Most early experiments tested drugs in transplanted tumour systems in mice. Often these bore little relationship to human disease. Recently more useful results have been obtained using the spontaneous AKR mouse leukaemia system. This closely corresponds to the clinical situation. Using this system it has been possible to study cell-cycle specific agents such as Ara C. This drug has been shown to be schedule-dependent. In other words, patient response to the drug depends critically on the timing of its administration. It is better to give 5-day courses of continuous Ara C therapy every

2 weeks, rather than protracted daily treatment. The spaced interruptions increase drug efficacy and allow bone marrow recovery.

The spontaneous AKR system has also been used to evaluate combination chemotherapy. In mouse lymphoma the best drug combination, with appropriate attention to schedule, has been cyclophosphamide, ara C, vincristine and prednisone. Experiments such as these may eventually enable us to modify and improve combination chemotherapy regimens in such conditions as Hodgkin's disease.

The above prediction systems have been developed mainly for the haematological malignancies. This has meant that drugs selected for clinical trials have tended to be most active in blood diseases. Results suggest that agents which are primarily antimetabolites are mostly cell-cycle specific. They have substantial activity in rapidly growing experimental leukaemias but limited activity in slowly growing solid tumours.

Increasing emphasis is now being placed on solid tumour models. Some of the newer drugs, particularly those which are not cell-cycle specific, are more active in solid tumours. These include the anthracycline antibiotics, actinomycin, bleomycin and especially cyclophosphamide and some of the nitrosourea derivatives.

2. Cytokinetics

Drugs act at different stages during the mitotic cycle. For instance, Ara C exerts its maximum effect during mitosis. By using a metaphase-arresting agent, such as vinblastine, it is possible to increase the efficacy of Ara C. Investigations indicate that if vinblastine is given 16 hours prior to Ara C, the cell-killing effect can be increased fourfold. Similar results have been obtained experimentally with bleomycin.

3. Chemical Structure

Advances in chemistry have made it possible to exploit observations on new drugs with greater rapidity and effectiveness. For instance daunorubicin was the first anthracycline antibiotic discovered. This drug is of some value in the treatment of acute myeloid leukaemia. However by making a slight modification to the hydroxal group in the 14th position, it was possible to produce Adriamycin. This slight difference in chemical structure resulted in a drug with a much better therapeutic index. Again the intercalation of these drugs with DNA is being investigated, and further modifications of the molecule based on biochemical rationale may yet be made.

4. Molecular biology

Perhaps one of the most exciting discoveries of the past few years was made by Temin and Baltimore. Working independently, they discovered simultaneously that the replication of RNA from the DNA template was a reversible phenomenon. Watson and Crick had originally suggested in their central dogma that this was a one-way process. Temin and Baltimore have now shown that RNA from certain tumour viruses is capable of transcribing its message on to DNA. The altered genome may then presumably render the cell neoplastic. The essential enzyme in this process is a reverse transcriptase. The intriguing possibility of inactivating this enzyme with such agents as rifampin and streptovaricin is being investigated.

There is also some evidence that certain large molecules may regulate cell proliferation and differentiation. Various inhibiting agents of these molecular factors have been identified. In one instance leukaemic cells in man were shown to be capable of differentiation. Formerly it was assumed that leukaemic cells must be destroyed. The above findings suggest that some normalization of the neoplastic process may yet be possible (Frei).

THE LYMPHOCYTE

In conclusion a word should be said about the development of the immune system and the discovery of two types of lymphocyte. Haematopoietic stem cells develop into erythrocytes, monocytes, platelets, granulocytes and lymphoid stem cells. In early life lymphocytes then develop into two different types, each of which plays an important role in the immune response and in the recognition between 'self' and 'non-self'. Those that pass through the thymus gland become T-lymphocytes and are responsible for cell mediated immunity. The others become B-lymphocytes and subsequently differentiate into plasma cells. The B-cells are responsible for immunoglobulin production and humoral immunity.

Although morphologically indistinguishable from each other at rest, important surface differences between T-cells and B-cells have been recognized on electron microscopy.

Several malignant disorders are now being tentatively reclassified in terms of T-cell disease and B-cell disease as shown in Table XV. Undoubtedly this will be revised and modified in the future.

TABLE XV

Lymphocyte malignancy

T-cell disease	B-cell disease
Hodgkin's disease	Multiple myeloma
Acute lymphoblastic leukaemia	Chronic lymphatic leukemia
Mycosis fungoides	Giant follicular lymphoma
	Burkitt's lymphoma

References

Burchenal, J., and Carter, S. K. *Cancer*, December, 1972, **30**, 1639.
Currie, G. A. *Eighty years of immunotherapy*, Brit. J. Cancer, 1972, **26**, 141.
D'Angio, G. *Cancer*, December 1972, **30**, 1528.
Frei, E. *Prospectus for Cancer Chemotherapy*, Cancer, December 1972, **30**, 1656.
Zubrod, C. G. *Cancer*, December 1972, **30**, 1474.

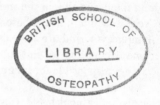

Index

abdomen, 91–3
absorption of radiation, 5
acoustic neuroma, 77
acromegaly, 79–81
actinomycin D, 19, 101, 156, 178, 182
adamantinoma, 59
adenoacanthoma, 126
adenoid cystic carcinoma, 71–3
adenolymphoma, 72
adenomas, pituitary, 79–81
adrenal tumours, 84
Adriamycin, 179, 188
aftercare, 32, 33, 39
afterloading, 170–1
Africa, radiotherapy, 48
age and treatment, 40
alcoholism, 50
Alkeran, 175
alkylating agents, 174–6
alpha particles, *18*, 168–9
alternate treatment days, 30
alveolar cell carcinoma, 85
alveolus,
    lower, 53–4
    upper, 54
amenorrhoea, 156, 162
amputation, 96
amyloidosis, 118
anaemia, 13, 29, 40
androgen therapy, 151
angiofibroma, 158
angiosarcoma, 101
ankylosing spondylitis, 160–1
antibiotics, 178–9
antimetabolites, 176–7
antrum, 55, 59, 60
anus carcinoma, 92–3
applicators,
    Fletcher-Bloedorn, 124; -Suit, 171
    strontium eye, *10*
    shell, 34

arabinosyl cystosine (Ara C), 179, 188
argentaffinoma, 85
arrhenoblastoma, 130
arsenical keratosis, 42
ascites, 131–2
asparaginase, 178
astrocytoma, 74–5
auto-immunity, 89
azathioprine, 164, 177

Bantus, carcinoma oesophagus, 87
basal cell carcinoma, 42–4
basophilic adenomas, 79–81
B-cells, 189
BCG, in melanoma, 47
BCNU, 180
beam direction shell, 34
Bence-Jones protein (BJP), 117, 119
benign disease, 160–5
Bergonie and Tribondeau, Law, 27–28
beta particles, see electrons
betatron, 3, 8, 169
betel nut chewing, 50
biopsy excision, 148, 150
bladder carcinoma, 139–43
bleeding, 38
bleomycin, 178–9
block dissection, 52
blood diseases, 112–9
bolus, 30
bone tumours, 95–9
    marrow damage, 13, 24
    metastases, 99
    necrosis, 58
boron capture therapy, 168
bowel, 24, 91–3
Bowen's disease, 42
Bragg-peak, 169

brain,
    abscess, 58
    metastases, 38, 78
    stem gliomas, 77
    tumours, 74–8
breast carcinoma, 146–53
    in pregnancy, 158
    male, 153
Brill-Symmers' disease, 109
bronchogenic carcinoma, see lung
    cancer
buccal mucosa, 56
Burkitt's lymphoma, 109–10
bursitis, 163
busulphan, 114, 176

caesium, 9, *10*
calcitonin, 82
californium, *11*
carcinoma-in-situ, 120, 124, 147
carotid haemorrhage, 55
cartilage necrosis, 44
cataract, radiation, 24, 70
cathetron, 171–2
CCNU, 180
cell,
    cycle, 17–18
    mammalian, 15
    morphology, 15, 28
    survival curve, 15–16
    synchrony, 19
    viable, 28
cell-cycle specific agents, 179, 187, 188
central nervous system
    damage, 23–4
    syndrome, 25
    tumours, 74–8
cerebellar tumours, 76, 78
cerebral tumours, 74–6
    oedema, 38
cervix carcinoma, 120–6
    in pregnancy, 159
chemodectoma, 58–9
chemotherapy,
    choice of, 182
    combination, 182–3
    dose, 182
    indications, 180
    length of, 182
    regional, 184
chest wall invasion, 147
childhood cancer, 154–9
chlorambucil, 115, 175

chondrosarcoma, 95–6
chordoma, 77–8
choriocarcinoma, 130, 132, 133
    male, 134
choroid melanoma, 46
chromophobe adenoma, 79–81
citrovorum rescue chemothrapy, 96,
    183
cobalt, 9, *10*
Codman's triangle, 95
colchicine, 180
colloid carcinoma, 147
colon carcinoma, 92
coma, 39
comedocarcinoma, 147
commando operation, 52
complications, see side effects
computer, 34
conical therapy, 88, *89*
conjunctiva melanoma, 46
cord, spinal compression, 39
corneal graft, 162
coronal arc, 80, *81*
corpus carcinoma, 126–8
craniopharyngioma, 79–81
curve, patient survival, 41
Cushing's disease, 79
cyclophosphamide, 110, 152, 156, 175,
    186
cylindroma, 59, 71–3, 147
cystadenocarcinoma, 130
cysteamine, 20
cysteine, 20
cytokinetics, 188
cytology, 121
Cytoxan, see cyclophosphamide

D_{37}, D_0, 16
damage,
    bone, 24
    eyes, 24, 159
    gonads, 25, 162
    intestinal tract, 24
    kidneys, 23
    lung, 23
    nerve, 23
    pregnancy, 158
    radiation, 12–13
    skin, 22
    whole body, 25
daunomycin, 156
daunorubicin, 188
dental care, 51–2

depth-dose curves, 9
dermatitis, radiation, 22
dermatofibrosarcoma, 101
deuterons, 169
di Guglielmos's syndrome, 112
di-methane sulphonates, 176
dose, 35–6, 40
dosimetry, 35
DNA, 15, 17–18
dual theory, 4
dysgerminoma of ovary, 130–2

ear, middle, 57–8
Ebstein-Barr virus, 109
ectropion, 44
elderly patients, 29, 36–7
electromagnetic radiation, 4
electrons, 8, 169–70
Ellinger's Law, 27
embryomas, 154–9
embryonal cell carcinoma, 134–6
emergencies, 38
endocrine therapy, 151
endometrial carcinoma, 126–8
endometroid carcinoma, 130
Endoxana, see cyclophosphamide
energy forms, 4
entropion, 44
eosinophilic adenoma, 79–81
eosinophilic granuloma, 110
ependymona, 75–6
epidermoid carcinoma skin, 42–4
epiglottis, 66
epilaryngeal, 66
epilation, 22, 26
epiphysis, 156
epithelioma, see skin cancer
Epodyl, 175
erythema, 22, 26
erythroplasia, see Querat
esthesio-neuroepithelioma, 61
ethmoid sinus, 59, 61
ethoglicid, 175
ethyleneimines, 175, 179
ethyl hydrazide of podophyllic acid, 19
eustachian tube, 63
Ewing's sarcoma, 96–7
exenteration, pelvis, 125
exposure, fatal, 26
external radiation beam, 30
extracorporeal irradiation, 164
extrapolation number (N), 16, 168
extrinsic larynx, 66–7

eye, 68–71
   benign conditions, 162
   radiation damage, 24

fauces, see tonsil
fibromas, 100
fibrosarcoma, 99–102
fibrosis, 22–3, 38
filters, compensating, 149
Finzi-Harmer fenestration, 65
floor mouth, 53
5-fluorouracil, 91, 177
foetus, see tonsil
follicular carcinoma, thyroid, 82–4
follow-up, 41
fractionation, 19–20, 35–6
fracture, pathological, 99
Frey's syndrome, 73
frontal sinus, 61
fungation, 38

ganglioneuroma, 84
gastric carcinoma, see abdomen
gastrointestinal injury, 24, 27, 91–3
gastrointestinal syndrome, 25
Gaucher's disease, 116, 163
genetic damage, 12, 25
giant cell tumour of bone, 97–8
giant follicular lymphoma, 109
gigantism, 79
gingiva, 53–4
glancing fields, 149
glioblastoma multiforme, 74–6
glioma, 74–7
globe of eye, 68
glomus jugulare, 57–9
glossopalatine sulcus, 55
glottis, 64-67
goitre, 82
gold, 80, 132
   implant, 51
   seeds, 33, 171
grade, histological, 40
graft rejection, 163–4
granuloma, malignant midline, 61–2
granuloma, orbit, 71
granulosa cell tumour, 130
Grenz rays, 162
growth deformity, 40, 154
gum, 53-54
gynaecomastia, 135, 145

haemangioblastoma, 78
haemangioma, 162-3
haematological syndrome, 23
haematuria, 38, 138, 140, 155
haemoptysis, 38, 65, 85
haemorrhage acute, 39
half-life, 10-12
half-value thickness, 6
Hand-Schuller-Christian disease, 110
hard palate, 54-5
Hassell's corpuscles, 90
hazards, see damage and side-effects
heavy chain disease, 117
heavy particle therapy, 168
hemianopia, 79-81
herpes simplex, 49
herpes zoster, 162
Heyman capsules, 127-8
histiocytosis X, 110-11
Hodgkin's disease, 103-7, 182
    pregnancy, 159
    thymus, 90
Honvan, 144
hormone therapy, 144, 151, 186
Hutchinson's syndrome, 157
hydatid mole, 133
hydrogen peroxide, therapy, 167
hydroxyurea, 19
hypercalcaemia, 118
hypernephroma, 138-9
hyperpituitarism, 79-81
hypersplenism, 116
hypertension, radiation induced, 23
hyperthyroidism, 164-5
hypopharynx, 66
hypophysectomy 79, 144, 152, 163
hypophysis, see pituitary
hypopituitarism, 79-81
hypothyroidism, 165
hypoxic therapy, 167

imidazole carboxamide, 180
immunoglobulin, 117, 164
immunological tolerance, 89
immunology, 158, 189
immunosuppression, 163-4
immunotherapy, 186-7
implants, see interstitial
Imuran, 164, 177
'Indian Club' radium needles, 93
infusion, 184
integral dose, 30

interstitial implants, 32-3, 51
    afterloading, 170-1
intracavitary irradiation, 31, 122-8
    afterloading, 170-1
intralobular carcinoma, 147
intramedullary tumours, 78
inverse square law, 6
inverted-Y therapy, 106
ionizing radiation, 5
iridium, 171
islet cell tumours, 84
isodose curves, 12
    construction, 34
    radium, 122
isotopes, see radioactive

kala azar, 116
Kaposi's sarcoma, 47-8
keloids, 161
keratoacanthoma, 44-5
kidney, 138-9

lacrimal gland, 69, 71
laparotomy, 105
large bowel cancer, 92
larynx, 64-7
lentigo malignum, 46
Letterer-Siwe disease, 110
leukaemia,
    acute, 116
    lymphatic, 114-16
    myeloid, 112-14
    radiation induced, 161
Leukeran, 175
leukoplakia, 42-3, 50, 65
Leydig cell tumours, 134
linear accelerator, 8
linear energy transfer (LET), 18-19,
    167-8
lip, 49-50
liposarcoma, 99-102
liver carcinoma, 92
localization, 34
lumpectomy, 148
lung carcinoma, 85-7
    damage, 23
    fibrosis, 23
    pneumonitis, 23
lymphangiosarcoma, 101
lymph node dissection, 50
lymphocytes, 89, 189

lympho-epithelioma, 62
lymphoma, 103–11
  abdomen, 91–92
  Burkitt's, 109
  cutis, 45
  hypersplenism, 116
  non-Hodgkin's, 103
  testis, 139
lymphosarcoma, 103–8
  antrum, 59, 103
  nasal fossa, 61
  orbit, 68–9
  thymus, 90

malabsorption syndrome, 39
malignant melanoma, 45–7, 68
mammography, 148
Manchester system, 122
mantle therapy, 105, *106*
mast cell disease, 111
mastectomy, 148
maxillary antrum, 55, 59, 60
maxillectomy, 60
maximum permissible dose, 13–14
mechlorethamine, 175
medullary carcinoma breast, 147
medullary carcinoma thyroid, 82–4
medulloblastoma, 75–7
  coma, 39
megavoltage, 8
melanoma, 45–7, 68
melphalan, 175
meningioma, 77
menopause, radiation induction, 162–3
6-mercaptopurine, 133, 177
mesonephroma, 130
metaphase arresting agent, 188
metastases, bone, 99
  brain, 38
methotrexate, 133, 176–7, 183
middle ear, 57–8
Mikulicz's disease, 73
mithramycin, 179
mitoclomine, 47, 180
mitomycin C, 179
mitotane, 180
mixed parotid tumour, 71–3
molecular biology, 188
MOPP therapy, 107, 183
moulds, 31, 44
  sandwich, 49
mouth care, 52

moving strip therapy, 35
mucoepidermoid carcinoma, 71–3
multihit and multitarget theories, 17
multiple fields, 30
multiple myeloma, 117–19
myasthenia gravis, 89, 90
mycosis fungoides, 45
Myeleran, see busulphan
myelitis, radiation, 24, 27
myeloproliferative disorders, 112, 119
myelosclerosis, 112, 119

nasal fossa, 61–2
nasopharynx, 55, 62–3
Natulan, see procarbazine
NDPP, 19
neck nodes, 50–52
  dissection, 66
  nodes fixed, 52
  retropharyngeal, 62
  unknown primary, 67
necrosis, bone, 58
nephroblastoma (Wilm's), 154–6
nerve, radioresistance, 23–4
neuroblastoma, 96–7, 156–8
neuro-fibrosarcoma, 100
neuropathy, carcinomatous, 78
neutrons,
  fast, *18*, 167–8
  slow, 168
nitrogen mustard, 175
nitrosourea, 180, 188
nominal standard dose (NSD), 21
non-Hodgkin's lymphoma, 103

oat-cell carcinoma, 85–7
oesophagus, 87–9
oestrogen therapy, 151
oligodendroglioma, 75–6
onchcytoma, 71
oophorectomy, 151
optic chiasma tumours, 77, 79–81
oral cavity, 49–56
orbit, 68–71
orbital exenteration, 60, 69
orchidectomy, 135
oropharynx, 63–4
osteoarthritis, 163
osteoclastoma, 97–8
osteolytic thrust, 98
osteonecrosis, 52

osteosarcoma, 95–6
otitis media, 57, 62, 63
ovary, carcinoma, 130–2
   transposition, 106
ovoids, 122
oxygenation, 37, 166
oxygen enhancement ratio (OER), 18,
   168
oxygen, hyperbaric, 142, 166, 167
oxyphil cells, 71

Paget's bone disease, 143
Paget's skin disease, 42, 147
pain relief, 38
pair reduction, 6
palate, hard and soft, 54–5
palatine arch, 55
palliation, 29, 38
Pancoast's syndrome, 86
pancreas carcinoma, 84, 92
Papanicolaou's smear, 121
papillary carcinoma thyroid, 82–4
para-follicular 'C' cells, 82
parallel opposed fields, 30
paraplegia, 99
Paris technique, 123
parotid, 71–3
Paterson-Parker rules, 31–2
pathological fracture, 99, 118
pediatric, see childhood
Pel-Ebstein, 104
penis carcinoma, 2, 136, 137
penumbra, 9
Peppard's syndrome, 157
peptic ulcer, 163
perfusion, 183–4
pericarditis, 39
perichondritis, 65
Peyronie's disease, 163
phaeochromocytoma, 82, 84
pharynx, 55–6, 66
phenylalanine mustard, 175
Philadelphia chromosome, 113
photo-electric effect, 6
photons, 5
pigmentation, 42
pinealomas, 84
pions, 168–9
pituitary ablation, see hypophysectomy
pituitary adenomas, 79–81
   pharyngeal wall, 55
   protons, 36

planning treatment, 33
plasmacytoma, 117–19
   extramedullary, 59, 61
Plummer-Vinson syndrome, 66, 87
points A and B, 122, 172
polycythaemia, 112–13
post-cricoid carcinoma, 66
post-herpetic neuralgia, 162
post-operative radiation, 37–8
prediction systems, 187
pregnancy and radiation, 158–9
pre-operative radiation, 36–8
procarbazine, 178
progesterone, 145, 152
prolactin, 80, 152
prostate carcinoma, 143–5
protection, 12
proton therapy, 80, 168–9
psychological factors, 29
pulmonary fibrosis, 83, 176
pulsed chemotherapy, 119
pyriform sinus, 66
pyrimethamine, 179

Querat, erythroplasia of, 42, 136, 137

rad, 7
radiation,
   dose, 35–6
   measurement, 7
   sources, 8
   supervoltage, 30
radioactive isotopes, 10–11, 33
   caesium, 9, 10
   cobalt, 9, 10
   gold, 33, 132, 171
   iodine, 164–5
   iridium, 10, 171
   phosphorus, 113, 132
   strontium, 10
   tantalum, 141
   yttrium, 11
radioactivity, 6
radiobiology, 15–21
radiomimetic drugs, 173
radioresistance 20, 28
radiosensitising agents, 19
radiosensitivity, 27, 36, 40
radium, 31–33
   implant, 93
   intracavitary, 122–8
   mould, 44

radon, 33, 51
rectum carcinoma, 92
recurrence, 41, 153
Reed-Sternberg cell, 104
relative biological effectiveness (RBE),
    8, 19, 168
rem, 8
renal pelvis tumours, 139
renal transplant, 163-4
residual disease, 41
results, 2, 40
respiratory obstruction, 39
ret, 21
reticulosis, see lymphoma
reticulum cell sarcoma, 96, 97, 108
retina, 69
retinoblastoma, 69-70
retromolar triangle, 55
reverse transcriptase, 189
rhabdomyosarcoma, 99-102
rheumatoid arthritis, 163
rifampin, 189
rodent ulcer, 42
roentgen, 7
rotation therapy, 30-31
round cell sarcoma, 96

sacrococcygeal chordoma, 77-8
salivary gland tumours, 71-3
sarcoma,
    botryoides, 101, 126
    soft tissue, 99-102
scattering, 5
scirrhous carcinoma, 147
schedule dependence, 188
Schiller's test, 121-2
scoliosis, 154
scrotal implantation, 135
scrotum carcinoma, 137
second primary, 41
seminoma, 134-6
sequestra bone, 58
serotinin, 20
sertoli cell tumour, 134
sex, 40
shoulder, cell survival curve, 17, 168
side effects,
    drugs, 2, 184-6
    radiation, 2, 39
simulator, 34
SI units, 14
sinuses, 59-61

sinusotomy, 60
Sjogren's syndrome, 73
skin,
    benign disease, 162
    cancer, 42-8
    damage, 22
    desquamation, 22
    necrosis, 22, 39
    sparing, 30
small bowel tumours, 91-2
smoking, lung cancer, 85
soft tissue tumours, 99-102
sparsomycin, 186
sphenoid sinus, 61-2
spheroidal carcinoma, 147
spinal cord depression, 39
spinal cord tumours, 78
spleen, irradiation, 114, 116, 119
splenectomy, 105
split-course therapy, 36-7
split-dose survival ratio, 17
squamous carcinoma, 42-4
staging, 40
sterility, 40
steroid therapy, 152, 186
stilboestrol, 144
Stockholm technique, 123
stomach carcinoma, 91
streptovaricin, 189
stridor, 39, 65
strip-field therapy, 35
strontium 90
    applicator, 10, 162, 164
stump carcinoma, 126
sub-glottic carcinoma, 64
sub-lethal damage, 17, 168, 185
superficial X-rays, 43
superior vena caval syndrome, (SVC),
    39
supraglottic carcinoma, 64
suprasellar tumours, 79-81
surgery and radiation, 37-8
synovial sarcoma, 100-1
syphilis, 43, 49, 50, 65, 136
syringomyelia, 160

tandems, 123-8
tantalum wire, 141
T-cells, 89, 189
tear duct stenosis, 44
teeth, 51-2
tenosynovitis, 163

teratoma, 130, 134–6
testis, 134–6
thecoma, 130
thermography, 147
thiotepa, 176
thiouracil, 20
thorax, 85–7
thrombocythaemia, 112
thymo-epithelioma, 90
thymus, 89–90
thyroid,
    cancer, 82–4, 89
    radio-iodine treatment, 10–11
thyrotoxicosis, 164–5
tissue equivalent material, 58
TNM staging, 40, 147
tongue, 52–3, 55
tonsil, 55–6
tonsillar fossa, 55–6
total nodal irradiation, 106
trachea, 89
transitional cell carcinoma,
    bladder, 140
    nasopharynx, 62
transvaginal therapy, 126
transverse myelitis, 58, 66
treatment planning, 33
tretamine (TEM), 176
trophoblastic tumours, 132
trunk bridge, 105
tubes, oesophageal, 88
tumour site, size, bed, 40

units, 51, 14
unknown primary, 67
ureter, 141

urethane, 179
urethra, 128, 129
uterus, see cervix, endometrium

vagina carcinoma, 128–9
Velban, see vinblastine
venereal disease, 136, see syphilis
vinblastine, vincristine (vinca-rosea
    alkaloids), 152, 156, 177, 188
vocal cords, 64–7
volume factor, 36–7, 41
vulva carcinoma, 129

Waldenstrom's macroglobulinaemia,
    117
Watkin's infusor, 184
wedge filters, 31, 31
Wertheim's hysterectomy, 125
Whartin's tumour, 72
whole-body radiation, 25, 113
Wilm's tumour, 154–6, 178
woodworker, antral carcinoma, 59

xerodema pigmentosum, 42
xerostomia, 39, 53, 73, 83
X-ray simulator, 34

yttrium, 11, 80, 137

zinc and castor oil ointment, 94
Zollinger-Ellison syndrome, 84